After Baby Comes

Rachel Taylor, RN

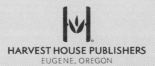

HARVEST HOUSE PUBLISHERS
EUGENE, OREGON

Published in association with The Blythe Daniel Agency, Inc., P.O. Box 64197, Colorado Springs, CO 80962-4197, www.theblythedanielagency.com.

Cover designer Faceout Studio, Elisha Zepeda
Interior designer Janelle Coury
Cover images © Marina Sidorova/Shutterstock

For bulk, special sales, or ministry purchases, please call 1-800-547-8979.
Email: CustomerService@hhpbooks.com

After Baby Comes

Copyright © 2025 by Rachel Taylor, RN
Published by Harvest House Publishers
Eugene, Oregon 97408
www.harvesthousepublishers.com

ISBN 978-0-7369-9048-6 (pbk)
ISBN 978-0-7369-9049-3 (eBook)

Library of Congress Control Number: 2024945655

Printed in Colombia

25 26 27 28 29 30 31 32 33 / NI / 10 9 8 7 6 5 4 3 2 1

To my mom.
You managed each day so well.
I am who I am because of your sacrifices.
Thank you.

Contents

Introduction: The Forgotten Trimester 7

Part 1: Frame

1. Perspectives and Expectation: Postpartum in
   Different Cultures 13
2. Prepping for Postpartum (It Isn't Too Late) 19
3. Your Physical Frame: The Why and
   How of Healing After Birth 27
4. Strengthening Your Body Again 41
5. C-Section Recovery 57
6. Breastfeeding 67

Part 2: Food

7. Postpartum Nutrition 87
8. Snack and Drink Recipes 95
9. Recipes for Nourishing Meals 99
10. Milk-Boosting Recipes 107

Part 3: Feelings and Fears

11. Connecting With Yourself Again 115
12. Postpartum Blues Versus Postpartum Depression 121
13. When Postpartum Breaks Your Brain 133
14. Overcoming Mom Guilt and Comparison Syndrome 141

Part 4: Faith

15. God of the Rocking Chair 149
16. What Is the One Thing You Don't Want to Forget? 155

Part 5: Family and Friends

17. Connecting Again in Your Relationship 161
18. Getting Back to the Bedroom 169
19. Boundaries, Balancing, and Dealing with Unwanted Help . . 177
20. How to Help Siblings and Pets Adjust 185
    Epilogue: Motherhood in Metamorphosis 191

Additional Resources

Help! My Baby Won't Stop Crying 195
Help! I'm Having Trouble Bonding with My Baby 197
When to Call My Healthcare Provider 199
Other Issues 201
A Note to the NICU Mama 203
A Note to the Mom of Multiples 205
A Note to the New Dad 207
Index 209
Notes 213

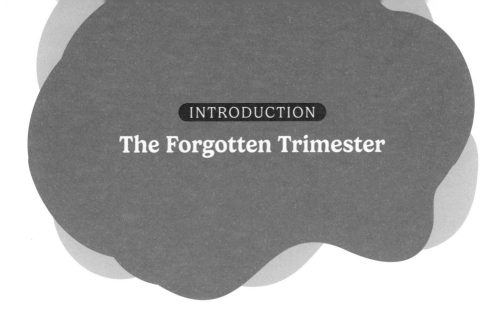

The Forgotten Trimester

Y ou are already a good mom.

Chances are you have been preparing for the arrival of your baby for months. You have read countless books, blogs, and social media posts on pregnancy, childbirth, breastfeeding, parenting, and more. You have probably done tons of research and read many reviews on the best baby products from highchairs to swaddles to car seats. And more than likely you have had some childbirth education, whether through a class at your local hospital or a baby book you ordered.

As a postpartum registered nurse, these are all the things I would want you to do before your baby comes. But one way I can help you prepare better for this pregnancy journey and after-baby experience is by providing you with a thorough resource for your fourth trimester. Many call this trimester *the forgotten trimester*, and unfortunately, at times, this has been the case. Studies show us that, during this trimester, postpartum moms feel their health concerns are not addressed,[1] that they are not being educated on what they need,[2] and they desire advice from healthcare professionals, not friends and family alone.[3] A healthcare team—OBGYNs, nurses, childbirth educators, and others—does a great job helping new mothers prepare for pregnancy, labor, delivery, and newborn care, but we have neglected the major transition that happens in the new mother's body, soul, and spirit during the many months following childbirth.

Just as being in labor and giving birth each have an emotional, physical, psychological, and spiritual aspect, I believe the postpartum period does as well. The term *postpartum* has become synonymous with postpartum depression, and yet the postpartum season is much more multifaceted. This limited mindset surrounding postpartum is unfortunate, because new moms need a holistic approach to all aspects of this time, not only the effects on a mother's mental health. Postpartum recovery needs to be more than an afterthought.

When I listened to one pediatrician educate a class of soon-to-be new parents, he said, "We have LDRP rooms which mean 'Labor, Delivery, Recovery'…and I forget what the other one is." Postpartum. I chuckled under my breath and thought, *How fitting. Isn't this the way it has been?* Of course, he is a wonderful pediatrician and a champion of new mothers. He simply had a long day in the office, and the word had just slipped his mind. But the lesson I took away was powerful.

We spend so much time preparing for pregnancy, labor, and birth, but postpartum education is at the most a 30-minute spiel. Most of us do not realize we should have been better prepared until we are already struggling in the days and weeks following the birth of our babies. Before I had my first baby, I felt I was well prepared for my postpartum journey and found myself shocked by the exhaustion, emotions, soreness, and recovery time I needed during those first few months after birth. It left me wondering, *How could I be a postpartum nurse and be so unprepared? What about other new mothers who did not have any experience with it?*

When that sweet, wonderful baby finally arrives, families shower the snuggly newborn with all their attention, while neglecting the mothers who brought those babies into the world. I am so sorry you are often overlooked because you, Mama, are important. What you are going through is important, and what you will continue to go through matters.

The Fourth Trimester

The fourth trimester is the term that refers to the first 12 weeks following childbirth. This idea was popularized more than 20 years ago by pediatrician Dr. Harvey Karp, who believes a baby's environment should be much like it was inside the mother's womb for the first three months following birth.[4] During this time, you and your baby are separate but still one. It is a time of great change, transition, and process not only in your baby, but also in you! And I'm here to help you through this season because as a nurse and a mom, I am confident that a healthy mother equals healthier motherhood.

Here you will find a judgment-free zone and a safe place to heal, recover, and process all that is happening in your newfound motherhood. Also, I will always promote a culture of honor here. I choose to honor hospitals, birth centers, obstetrics, midwifery, and doulas. Each brings unique assets to the table, and I believe there is room for all. When we can honor each other, we will be able to work as a team and benefit new mothers.

We are going to learn to ditch perfectionism and comparison and embrace our own process and motherhood journey. In these pages, you will find evidence-based, practical advice for your recovery that is proven and effective, and you will be guided in what to expect throughout these first three months. You'll also learn when it is time to reach out for help. I have pulled in several experts on pelvic floor physical therapy, body work, lactation, and even relationships to help in every area of our lives in the fourth trimester. Drawing from my professional experience, I have also developed and placed Nurse's Tips for you throughout the book to offer you important help and reminders along the way.

Though some do not acknowledge the difficulties of the fourth trimester, others describe it as revolutionary. It is a time of detailed, focused, internal process and work, much like a metamorphosis. We are changing on the inside even more than on the outside. As the caterpillar changes into a butterfly, it goes through an intense, dark process. Parts of itself fade as other parts that have been inside emerge. These then develop into many more new and beautiful parts until one day it breaks from the cocoon and soars into the sky.[5] I can't imagine the process is all pleasant, but the results are beautiful. This is motherhood—a glorious transition of who you once were into a new, more beautiful version of you.

Mama, you are about to embark on the most life-changing thing you will ever do. Becoming a mother is hard and wonderful all at the same time. You will love more than you ever thought possible, and you will wonder how you ever did life without this child. You may feel incredibly anxious and scared. And at other times, you may feel like you are a complete failure. If I were sitting right beside you, I would reach over, place my hand on yours, and say, "Every single thing you will feel is okay. In fact, it is good because it means you are a new mom experiencing all the emotions and feelings that moms do."

Allow yourself to experience it all—the triumphs, failures, challenges, and glory that motherhood contains. I am here to be a guidepost for you and share with you what this passage into your fourth trimester holds for your physical, emotional, and spiritual healing and recovery. I bring over a decade of experience working with thousands of brand-new mothers, just like you, and I hope to make this journey a bit easier for you. Please know you are surrounded by so many others who have gone through what you have, and you are not alone.

As a postpartum nurse for more than 15 years, I can finally say, now you can take your nurse home with you. So, let's get started. I am so glad you are here!

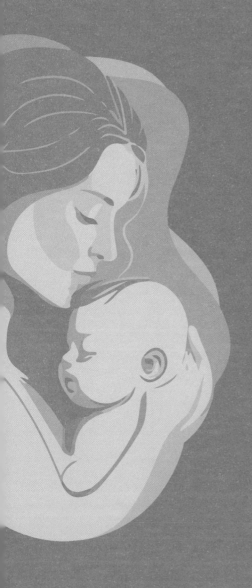

PART 1

Frame

CHAPTER 1

Perspectives and Expectations: Postpartum in Different Cultures

B irth is universal, but the *recovery* from birth is highly cultural.
I learned this early in my nursing career when I cared for an Asian patient who chose only to eat warm foods following the birth of her baby. Her husband explained to me that this was common in their culture. Postpartum mothers would solely eat warm foods, drink warm drinks, and take warm baths.[1] She bundled up in warm clothes and kept hot packs close by. This was comforting to the mother and is believed to help with *chi*, a positive energy moving through the body that promotes healing and comfort. For 40 days, the mother's support system took care of everything for her. Her jobs were to rest, nurse, and bond with her baby.

Working hard to be culturally aware, one of my fellow nurses, Katie, went into one of her patients' rooms to introduce herself. Her patient, who had a Hispanic background, was standing beside her bed. Katie, eager to learn, excitedly exclaimed, "Is this a cultural thing?" The patient giggled and said, "No, my bottom hurts when I lay down." Katie and her patient laughed and laughed over the conversation. These two stories remind us that there are universal postpartum experiences, such as discomfort in the bottom, and then there are others that depend on your location around the globe.

If I were to travel to Australia as a postpartum nurse caring for patients, I might hear the common phrase "wetting the baby's head." My American nursing perspective would cause me to assume the parents were discussing washing their baby's hair. Instead, it means having a drink to honor the newest member of the family. This is a common tradition in Europe as well. Australians also commonly stock the freezer full of meals for the parents of a brand-new baby. (A big-time yes to this tradition please!)

In Belgium and France, pelvic floor health is a big focus, and insurance covers around 20 visits to be used before birth and in postpartum with the option of receiving more if needed. The most common postnatal care is focused around pelvic floor recovery for the mother.[2] These cultures understand the importance of pelvic floor health and how this area can affect a woman—either positively or negatively—for the rest of her life.

In Nepal, women recover in their in-laws' homes for at least ten days. During this time, new mothers may not eat salt or green vegetables, bathe, or go out in the sun. Birth is considered unclean, and a mom must undergo certain rituals and allow a certain number of days to pass to be considered clean again. After ten days, the birth mother may go to her own parents' home. A mustard oil massage is then given to both mom and baby to relax the muscles and smooth the joints.[3]

Many cultures, such as in Colombia and other Latin American countries, observe a 40-day practice. This is a time when care is focused on supporting the mother and allowing her to rest and bond with her baby. The support system cooks meals, cares for other children, and takes care of household chores.

In the United States, a typical postpartum recovery looks like staying two days in the hospital (three to four if the mother had a cesarean section) and a follow-up visit at six weeks postpartum. Friends and family may bring meals to help the new parents, and visitors come to meet the new baby. Postpartum care tends to be focused on the baby, but more professionals are beginning to recognize the need for better new-mother support.

Postnatal retreats are on the rise in certain parts of the world.[4] Mothers can be fully pampered with massages and professional baby help while they rest. This sounds like a dream for most of us! Unfortunately, it will more than likely remain a dream because of the high cost. Even those who can afford it might prefer at-home, sustainable support as opposed to a one-night respite.

Many cultures practice rituals for the placenta, and there are several different disposal methods including discarding it as medical waste, burying it, incineration, placing it in a specific area (like underneath a tree), or eating it. In ancient Egypt, the placenta was believed to be the baby's guardian angel.[5]

Today, the placenta is treated differently around the world. In Chinese and Japanese culture, it is common to bury the placenta. In Bali, it is normal practice to place the placenta in a coconut and hang it from a tree in the village graveyard. This is believed to protect the baby from sickness and misfortune.[6] In Ukraine, a midwife buries the placenta anywhere except where it may be stepped on. It is believed that if someone were to step on it, it would make the mother infertile.[7]

Is there a right way to recover from birth? Perspective and expectations play a huge role in our postpartum recovery. If we have a baby in Latin America, we may have a less anxious postpartum experience because we know we will have support from women who have been through what we have been through. We might expect help with meals, housework, and other children because this is normal in our culture. It would be common to anticipate several weeks of rest.

If we give birth in the United States, we may be under the impression that postpartum is a breezy experience. With a two-day recovery period and a single six-week follow-up visit where most of us get the "all-clear to go back to pre-pregnant life," we may get the false impression that that is all there is to it. I know I did, and I was a postpartum nurse!

It is not a secret that postpartum can be tough. Mom influencers all over the world discuss the challenges of this season. And even celebrities who have plenty of financial resources to hire help speak out about its difficulties.

Even though in recent years, much attention has been given to how hard postpartum is, I think it is just as important to look at *why* it can be such a challenge and *how* to improve our experience in the fourth trimester. This takes a multifaceted approach.

We are complex, multidimensional creations made up of three parts: spirit, soul, and body. I believe it is nearly impossible to affect one part of us without affecting the other. I think this is one reason we cannot take a "do this and this, and you will be great" approach. Anything that affects our bodies the way birth and having a newborn does is sure to affect our emotions, our mental health, our relationships, and our faith.

But I have wonderful news! Postpartum is not a ship on fire where those who survive emerge from the ashes traumatized and smelling of smoke. It is a journey of authenticity that gives us the opportunity to transform into the most whole version of ourselves that we have ever been. We are not meant to go back to our pre-pregnancy state. We are meant to experience a metamorphosis into more of who we are as women and as mothers.

In the following chapters, you will find a roadmap for embracing the metamorphosis taking place in the postpartum season, overcoming the challenges, and healing more effectively in every area of your life. From breastfeeding to pelvic floor health, to emotional and mental wellness, all the way to connection and communication issues that can come up in marriage, you will find a wholeness guide to help you have the best fourth trimester you can have.

Feel free to skip around to the topics you need when you need them. I wrote this book for that very reason. Let's be honest: It is so easy to grab the phone and google questions at two o'clock in the morning and suddenly find we are down a deep rabbit hole of information that produces more anxiety. I do not want that for you!

I hope to bring a better understanding of all that a new mother experiences after birth, so you find the grace you need to engage the process, heal better, and enjoy the journey. Let's venture into this postpartum season of life together. Welcome to your newfound motherhood.

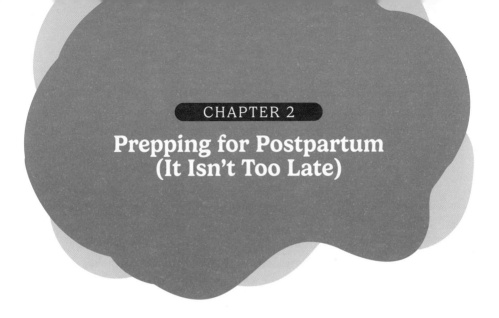

CHAPTER 2

Prepping for Postpartum (It Isn't Too Late)

Two days before my due date, I waddled into the La-Z-Boy store to purchase a rocking chair. Up and down and up and down we went as we tried out all the options. One of the sales associates looked at my husband and me and said, "The most important question is who will be doing most of the rocking?" We stared at each other blankly for a few moments, until I spoke up and said, "Probably me."

It never occurred to us that we needed to discuss what our roles and expectations would be for when our baby arrived. We had done the things we were told: We went to prenatal appointments, made a registry, had the showers, put together the baby's room. Weren't we ready?

If you have not birthed your baby yet, a month before your due date is still a great time to start preparing. Have open and honest conversations with your spouse and ask each other questions about roles and expectations now. The more you understand each other's expectations, the more you can meet those and navigate conflicts that creep up once your baby comes. Even if you have birthed your baby already, I'll share some great conversation starters that will help determine ownership, roles, and expectations.

You may even want to go as far as making an Our Growing Family mission statement. This should be simple, just a sentence or two, and include the most important things to you both. Mine looks something like this: "Love well. Choose connection over fear." The conversations and choices you make should always reflect your mission statement. This practice comes from Steven Covey and totally changed how we operate in my family.[1] If you need help creating a mission statement, there are great resources online.[2]

In the medical community, we have a phrase we say when emotions are high, situations are chaotic, and we need to refocus on what matters in the moment. It reminds us that we are working as a team. We all know if someone states, "Do you hear that helicopter?" we need to refocus. And it works! No need for yelling or gesturing. Every person responds without alarming the patient. It also builds trust between everyone in the room, including the patient.

If a doctor yells at a nurse or a nurse curses at another nurse, this degrades trust because it looks like we do not value each other. It is completely uncomfortable to witness a conflict that includes disrespect. The same is true in other relationships. If we are struggling in the postpartum period and we are yelling at each other, waving our arms, pointing the finger, using passive-aggressive language, or even giving the silent treatment and stonewalling, we are not heading toward success.

Because of this, I recommend you and your significant other negotiate a phrase you can both use when tensions are high or you simply don't know how to ask for what you need, but you know you need something.

My husband and I use "finger guns" at each other when we need to talk privately. Not only is this quick, but it also adds an aspect of humor that alleviates the situation when we see the other finger gunning. There is always a *pew-pew-pew* noise that goes along with it.

A phrase or signal can really be anything as long as it is meaningful to you both and you will recognize it as a cue to stop and listen. Make an agreement between you that if this phrase is spoken, you give the other your immediate attention. Watching TV, gaming, or scrolling on your phone needs to pause right away, because the other person is your priority in this moment.

When I caught up with one of Birmingham, Alabama's most sought-after doulas, Jeanna McNeil, I asked her, "What is the one place you see most new parents struggle with in postpartum?" She responded, "I feel that when it comes to postpartum, many families enter into it vastly under-prepared. I think that there's often such an emphasis on preparing for the birth that postpartum preparations sort of fall by the wayside. And while acquiring education and resources for birth is absolutely imperative, it is equally important for the postpartum season as well." [3] I completely agree. The amount of rest needed, healing, recovery, emotions, hormone changes, and changes to the relationship dynamic is a surprise for many.

NURSE'S TIP

Stock up on hand sanitizer and antibacterial soap. You will use these often as you care for your baby.

Roles and Responsibilities

As promised, here are some conversation starters for couples to help them determine who does what in the coming days.

Who Is Feeding the Baby at Night?

If mom is exclusively breastfeeding, will dad commit to be on diaper-changing duty or putting-baby-back-to-sleep duty? If mom is pumping or formula feeding, do we agree to take turns warming bottles and feeding at night? Or maybe we switch out nights, so we each get longer turns of uninterrupted sleep.

Who Changes Diapers?

Let's be honest, it is probably both of us. But it is an important conversation to have. I have taken care of one parent or the other who was so disgusted by diaper changes that they were unable to do it without getting sick. If this is the case in your home, what is the plan?

Who Runs to the Store for Essentials When We Are Suddenly Out?

It is bound to happen. We realize that we are down to one diaper or that we just used the very last baby wipe. Does dad want to run down the road or does mom want to get out for a bit to get some fresh air?

Who Is Doing What Chores?

Chore assignments may need to be reevaluated in the first several weeks after delivery. Depending on how birth went, a mom may be unable to do much more than walk around for over a month. This is not laziness! It is the sign of a body that is in need of longer recovery. If this is the case, who is doing laundry? Who is getting dinner on the table? Who is starting the dishwasher? How are we keeping the household running smoothly?

Hopefully these questions spurred you to think of some others that would relate to your own situation. The more we communicate our expectations and roles, the less conflict we will find ourselves in when the situation comes up.

Even once a plan is agreed upon, choose to be flexible. If you know he had a horribly long day at work and a huge presentation coming up the following day, offer to take some extra duties for him. He should do the same for you. Or even ask a family member or dear friend to pitch in for the night.

Truthfully, marriage is so much more than 50/50. It is days of picking up the slack when your spouse simply can't. It is giving more than you receive on some days, and then receiving more than you give on others.

Who Is on Your Team?

The priority in the immediate postpartum period is physical recovery, learning to nurse, bonding with your baby, and resting. You will need support during this time, but it is important to consider who will fit the bill.

> ### NURSE'S TIP
>
> A rolling cart is a convenient and helpful way to keep supplies in reach and is easily transferrable between rooms. Stock with snacks, water, hair ties, breastfeeding supplies, and baby products. For specific product recommendations, visit Amazon.com/Shop/MamaDidItOfficial

Recovery from birth is an intimate time. I am consistently in awe that I have been privileged to be a part of so many recoveries (a big thank-you to each mama who trusted me with their care!). The first couple of weeks after birth continue to be an intimate time and should be valued as such. Your body is healing, your breasts are leaking, your schedule is turned on its head, and you are caring for a newborn. Bottom line, you are now a new mother.

Dividing your support system into three groups can be helpful. You have probably already had conversations about how to handle *that* person or what to do about visitors. Think on who you could place in these groups and gracefully communicate with them ahead of time.

Group 1: The Team

Think of these as the "maids of honor" of the birth world. They are available for the first three weeks after you give birth. They understand you need lots of time with your baby. They are not there only to hold the baby (it is a bonus if they get to). Your job is to care for your baby, and their job is to care for you. They will do housework, laundry, make you padsicles, bring you lactation cookies, set up sitz baths, feed your pet, play with other children, or arrange dinner for you. This could be a mom, a sister, a mother-in-law, a best friend, or a postpartum doula. Communicate to this group ahead of time and ask, "Would you be able to help me recover by taking care of things so I can rest and bond with my baby?" Asking if they will do a specific task (or two or three) will help them know exactly how to meet that need.

Group 2: The Weekenders

Present three weeks after birth, these are the "bridesmaids" of postpartum. These are those who may not be as helpful but are loved ones. They still should not be people you feel the need to entertain—this is out of the question. You are still recovering! They get to meet the baby, hold the baby, and bring a meal if they offer. Take advantage of these visits by asking them ahead of time if they mind holding the baby while you shower or take a nap. Most of them will be thrilled to say yes! Communicate to this group and let them know: "We will need about three weeks to rest and recover but then look forward to visits."

Group 3: The Community

From six weeks on, these people are similar to "wedding guests." You mingle and have conversations with them when the time is right, either in your home or out and about. These are your mommy friends or your community groups. Meetings with these people help you find your voice again. You will be able to share struggles and encourage one another in your new roles. You will not worry so much if your baby cries or needs to nurse because these people are in the same season of life as you. A new mom's small group from church, a neighborhood group, a mommy-and-me exercise class, or a lactation support group can fit this need if you feel lonely in this season. It is also a great way to be a friend and build new friendships.

It is a lot of work to get you and your new baby ready and out of the house, but it is worth it. You will feel better emotionally and more like yourself after your outing.

It does not matter how much you love someone. If they are degrading you as a mother, criticizing what you do, or puffing themselves up by putting you down, they do not need to be part of your support group. You can find more on these situations in chapter 19.

QUESTION:
What size clothes will I need postpartum?

ANSWER: Though your uterus is back to normal size by six weeks postpartum, your body will continue to change for several months. In the fourth trimester it is important to have on hand three to four outfits that fit well and you feel confident in. These outfits can be as simple as leggings, a nursing tank, and a long flannel shirt or a maxi dress. Don't try to cram yourself in pre-pregnancy clothes too soon. It isn't worth it!

For Those Who Offer to Help

Have one of your baby shower hostesses or even someone who offers to be helpful arrange a meal train for you once your baby is born. There are websites devoted to making this easier![4] Having meals show up at your door is such a blessing in the early days after birth. The person organizing the meal train can also set boundaries for you ahead of time, if you wish, by adding notes or an email that says something like, "Please be aware that mom and baby are recovering and need rest. Plan to keep visits to ten minutes. They will be ready for longer visits in three weeks." Most people will have no trouble understanding!

If meal train dinners book up quickly, ask for a few days' worth of bento box lunches. Items like chicken salad, fresh fruits, nuts, cheeses, wraps, and salads with dressing on the side are a great way to care for a new mother. How easy is it when those hunger pangs hit to simply walk to the fridge and grab a box? Also, be sure to inform the helper of allergies or dietary preferences.

A protein basket is another favorite among new mamas. A basket full of things like healthy protein bars, grass-fed beef sticks, crackers, trail mix, and nuts is a great gift for a new mom. Add a treat or two for fun. Breast-feeding mothers need an extra 500 calories every day, and this is an easy way for her to remember to get those calories in.

• • • • • • • • • • •

Why prep so much before birth? We tend to greatly underestimate our needs in the fourth trimester. Of course, things you didn't prepare for will come up along the way, but doing what you can ahead of time will calm anxieties, ease tension, and help you navigate the waters of postpartum a bit easier.

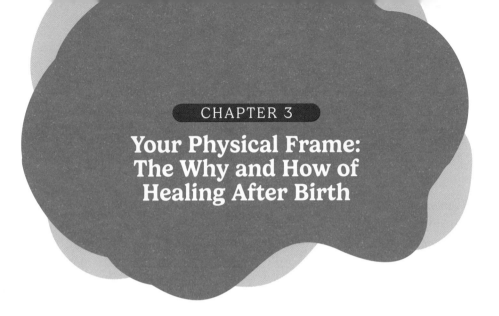

CHAPTER 3

Your Physical Frame: The Why and How of Healing After Birth

I t was 1:15 a.m., and my firstborn was finally here. Cries pierced the early June morning. I stared at him for hours as my nurses worked around me, putting me back together after the delivery of my baby boy.

It was around 7 a.m. when I finally dozed off for the first time. I awoke 30 minutes later to the nurse checking my baby's temperature and taking my vital signs. Now it was time to breastfeed again. *Oh well*, I thought, *I'll catch up on sleep eventually*. I had my baby in my arms and the hard part was over.

Well, not quite.

Pregnancy and childbirth are challenging, and we discount how long it will take to heal and recover from these changes to our bodies. Our days in the birthing center or hospital are only the beginning of a journey that will take us months to travel.

Chances are we feel pretty good immediately after delivering our babies, although exhaustion can be normal too. Labor may last hours or, for some, days. Some mamas experience medical interventions or cesarean sections that were not anticipated. And by the time our baby is skin-to-skin on our chest, our body has gone through one of the biggest transitions it will ever go through in our lives.

The brain literally changes during pregnancy, birth, and the postpartum period. It is not simply a theory that motherhood changes us. It is science. Research has proven that, during this time, our brains are experiencing "brain plasticity," where they are reformatting more than they are at any other time in our lives.[1] They are eliminating old connections while facilitating new ones, which may also be part of the reason we are more vulnerable to mental health issues such as postpartum depression and anxiety.[2] And it may be at least one of the reasons we experience "mommy brain" (also called "placenta brain"). *Mommy brain* is the term used to describe the way we might feel hazy or suddenly forget things. In other words, there is a good reason we put the milk in the cabinet.

These research findings on our changing brains were consistent for all new mothers regardless of their life experiences. But it should also be noted that these changes did not only cause disruptions or unwanted behaviors in the mother. It is also believed that our brains reorganize in this way to assist us with all the new priorities we will have. Studies show these changes help us bond with our baby, teach us how to make their needs our priority, and help us focus on caring for them.[3] In other words, it helps us make the transition to being mama.

·········COMMON POSTPARTUM SYMPTOMS·········

Hair Thinning: During pregnancy, hair shedding slows down. Now the body makes up for that.

Night Sweats: Caused by low estrogen and the body getting rid of extra fluid from pregnancy.

Shoe Size Change: Pregnancy hormones relax the ligaments in our feet, causing the bones to widen and spread.

Vision Change: The extra fluid in pregnancy can cause changes to the shape and thickness of our corneas.

As much as our brains change, our hormones are not too far behind. Following the birth of our babies, it is normal for endorphins to be at high levels. This increase helps us cope with the process of birth, and may make us feel alert, attentive, and possibly even euphoric at birth.[4] This is one of the reasons we see new moms go for hours or even days on little sleep and still feel fairly normal. It is also normal for us to feel emotionally weepy as these endorphins and other hormones like progesterone begin to decrease. We may find ourselves crying but we're not sure why. The hormone changes can also cause the new mother to have night sweats. It is not abnormal for us to wake up in the night with soaking wet pajamas from all the sweating.

While some hormones are dropping, others like oxytocin and prolactin are rising.[5] Oxytocin causes contractions during labor. It also causes "after-birth pain," which is the cramping we will feel in our uterus for several days following birth. This helps our uterus stay contracted and return to its original size. Oxytocin has also been called "the bonding hormone," as it promotes a special bond between mom and baby. As baby nurses, oxytocin is released, which promotes bonding, and also causes contractions in mom's uterus, which speeds healing and aids to prevent postpartum hemorrhage. (Aren't our bodies amazing?) Prolactin encourages breast-milk production and also helps with the mother-baby bond. Everything within us is making way for the ability to sustain and care for our new baby.

QUESTION:
Should I be cramping so much after birth?

ANSWER: Cramping after birth is from the process of involution, also called *after-birth pains*. These contractions are stronger when breastfeeding and get stronger after each birth. You may notice an increase in bleeding with the cramps. All this is your uterus working to expel blood and shrink back to its original size. It lasts two to three days.

Here I want to pause and bring to your attention the drastic number of changes you have already gone through just a few days postpartum. Now is a great time to learn to be kind and give yourself grace. When you feel tempted to blame yourself for not handling things as you expected, for being too emotional, or if you think you are not healing or adjusting the way other moms seem to, remember this process is not a walk in the park. This is a metamorphosis journey of your brain, your hormones, and your life. Even if we remove the fact that you now have a new baby plus everything caring for a newborn entails, an incredible amount has changed on the inside of you. Your brain, hormones, and body have been and still are going through enormous transitions. And on top of that, you are sustaining a new baby. Be kind to yourself, Mama. It is only fair.

Two days after birthing my first baby, I was about to be discharged from the hospital. I sheepishly turned to my nurse and said, "I know I do this for a living, but my bottom really hurts. Could you please just check it and make sure I don't have a hematoma (blood that collects in the tissues around the perineal area) or something?" She of course obliged, and said, "Nope, everything looks good."

Are you kidding me? I thought, *How is this normal?* My heart immediately went out to every new mother I had ever cared for. You don't know until you know.

It is true that discomfort comes after having a baby. But there are also ways you can greatly help with the pain and help your body heal better. Because I was unaware of how birth would affect me, I put way too many expectations on myself to feel good once I got home. Recovery is certainly a process.

QUESTION:
How long should I use cold therapy on my perineum?

ANSWER: Chandler Harris, midwife (LM, CPM), states, "I recommend cold therapy for the first 24 hours after birth to help with inflammation. After that, warmth is best to promote blood flow and healing to the area. Ice packs or padsicles can also be used as the mother feels she needs it to help soothe the area."[6]

Once the first week after birth passed by, I felt ready to go to my Walmart Superstore. I was moving around well at home, so I would move around well in the store…I thought. I pushed my cart all the way to the back of the store and realized I had made a big mistake. Leaning on the buggy for support, I turned around, pushed it back outside, and went home.

Every mom's recovery may look a bit different because every mom's birth is a bit different. A mom who pushed for three hours may be sorer than a mom who pushed for 30 minutes. She's liable to feel soreness in muscles she forgot she even had! A mom who had a first-degree tear will heal quicker than a mom with a fourth-degree. The degree of tears and episiotomies (an incision made during birth to widen the vaginal opening) ranges from one to four, with four being the most severe.

Remember to take your birth story into account when learning what you need and when. I encourage resting as much as possible for at least the first two weeks. No running errands, cooking meals, doing laundry, cleaning, or other chores if you can help it. This is all you should do in a day: rest, eat, drink, shower, and care for your baby (more on this in chapter 4). And there are good reasons for this intentionally slower pace.

Your cervix is continuing to close and heal for around six weeks, along with the wound your placenta left in your uterus. As your uterus shrinks, so does the wound. (Did you know that breastfeeding speeds this process up?) If you had stitches because of a tear or episiotomy, these are healing for several weeks and may cause some itching as they dissolve. You may even pass a thread or two onto your pad as they heal.

If you pushed for any amount of time, you probably have some hemorrhoids. Witch hazel pads, hydrocortisone cream, or lidocaine cream can offer relief. These get better in time, but sitting straight down may be out of the question for several weeks. I had a visitor come to see my baby and noticed I was carefully lowering myself down on the edge of my couch while sitting on a hip. She removed my pillows and said, "Go ahead, sit on down. Get comfortable." I modestly said, "I can't." With a tear that's healing plus hemorrhoids from pushing a baby out, effortlessly sitting down was a no-go.

NURSE'S TIP

If it feels uncomfortable to sit straight down after birth, try sitting on a curved breastfeeding pillow, like the Boppy pillow. This keeps pressure off your perineum and makes sitting down easier.

Sitz Baths

Sitz baths are another game changer for the sore perineum (the area between the vagina and anus). They decrease inflammation, are soothing, and, with certain ingredients, can also be healing to the area.[7] You will probably be quite sore in your vagina, perineum, and bottom for several weeks, especially the first week. Using a perineal squirt bottle and touching the area as little as possible is a must as you heal. This also helps prevent infection.

SOOTHING SITZ BATH RECIPE

¼ cup dried comfrey leaves
½ cup dried lavender flowers

¼ cup dried rosemary leaves
¼ cup fine grain Himalayan pink salt

¼ cup dried calendula flowers

1. Combine all the ingredients and store until ready to use. Bring two quarts of water to a boil. Add one ounce (about a handful) of dried herbs, and steep for 20 minutes. Strain the herbs out of the water, and keep the liquid. Can be stored in the fridge for up to four days.

2. Pour three cups into a sitz bath basin. Fill the rest of the way with water. Make sure the temperature is comfortable. Sit for 15 minutes.

For the first week, I recommend a goal of one sitz bath per day. If making your own sitz bath recipe sounds too overwhelming, you can try a premade product like Earth Mama Organic Herbal Sitz Bath.

Perineal Care

Each time you change your pad, use your perineal bottle to squirt off from front to back. In the first 24 hours after birth, I recommend ice packs with pad changes. After 24 hours, incorporate warmth to the area and use a padsicle, icepack, lidocaine cream, or Dermoplast Postpartum Spray (with the blue lid) as needed for soothing the area. Rachel Moran, pelvic floor physical therapist, recommends that new moms use gel ice packs for the perineum. These ice packs are reusable and better conform to a mom's body than the disposable variety, and can further cut down on swelling and inflammation. Never use a padsicle/ice pack and Dermoplast/lidocaine at the same time! Always rotate these products. Not doing so can cause damage to your skin tissue.

DIY PADSICLES

15 overnight maxi pads	12 oz. alcohol-free witch	lavender essential oil
3-inch cotton rounds (45)	hazel with aloe (like Thayers)	gallon-sized storage bags (2)

METHOD

1. Open the bottle of witch hazel and add five drops of lavender essential oil to the bottle. Swirl to mix.

2. Place the cotton rounds into a large bowl, and pour the witch hazel over the top.

3. Gently unfold 15 maxi pads and line with three witch hazel pads each.

4. Fold each pad back up, wrap in the original wrapper, and place the pads in the gallon storage bags. Freeze until ready to use.

5. After cleaning perineum, use as you would a maxi pad.

Can be made two weeks ahead of due date.

Urinating

You may notice that peeing for the first week may make your urethra (the passageway from your bladder to the outside—in other words, your pee hole) sting. A low percentage of moms experience a small tear at their urethra during birth. This can take several weeks to heal and may cause burning when peeing as well. To relieve this, use your perineal squirt bottle and squirt the area with warm water *as* you urinate. It works! Stinging at the beginning of urination after having a baby is normal, but experiencing pain the entire time you pee could be signs of an infection. Let your provider know if peeing hurts the whole time.

If you find it hard to empty your bladder, try breathing in peppermint essential oil or dropping a few drops into the toilet. Leaning forward while sitting on the toilet can also help you fully empty your bladder. You may also notice that you start and stop peeing several times before finishing. Inconsistent urine stream is normal at first when your bladder is recovering, but if it continues past a few days, let your healthcare provider know.

HOW TO MAKE THE FIRST POOP EASIER

Stay hydrated.

Slowly introduce fiber-friendly foods like oatmeal.

Take stool softeners or magnesium oxide until regular.

Use a potty stool or elevate your knees above your hips.

Don't strain. Let gravity help.

Bleeding

Though we do not have periods in pregnancy, we get to make up for some of that bleeding once our baby is born. Lochia, the bleeding you have after birth, lasts from three to six weeks. It is *not* a period, but the bleeding pattern can behave similarly. For instance, it begins as a heavy flow and moves to a lighter one. Lochia starts out red and changes to brown, then yellow and white. Also, lochia may even skip a day before it completely goes away. Watch your bleeding, though. If your bleeding increases at home, it is a sign you are pushing yourself too hard. Take it easier.

If you are soaking a pad in one hour, call your doctor. Losing that amount of blood so quickly could be a sign of postpartum hemorrhage. Signs of postpartum hemorrhage include passing large, baseball size clots, soaking a maxi pad in one hour, dizziness, passing out (or almost), pale skin, and a fast heartrate. This is not anything to play around with. If you experience any of these symptoms, call your healthcare provider immediately.

QUESTION:
Should I encapsulate my placenta?

ANSWER: Current research tells us that ingesting your placenta offers similar effects as a placebo. However, mothers all around the world would say differently. Claimed benefits include fewer incidents of postpartum depression, better hormonal balance, and quicker recovery in the presence of postpartum hemorrhage. Bottom line: More research is needed to confirm or reject this practice.[8]

First Period

When your first period will return varies from woman to woman and greatly depends on whether you breastfeed or are formula feeding. A mama who formula feeds may get her first period by six weeks postpartum. A breastfeeding mama will get her first period anywhere from a few months in to over a year after birth. Some women have a lighter period the first go-round, and others experience heavy bleeding with lots of cramping. Either can be totally normal. Usually the longer you breastfeed, the more delayed your period is, but breastfeeding is *not* a form of birth control. At some point you will ovulate and be unaware of it. When this happens, you can become pregnant again.

Your healthcare provider will discuss birth control options at your six-week follow-up visit. Typically, it is much easier to get pregnant once you have been pregnant, especially during the fourth trimester. Your body is like, "Been there, done that, know what to do!" Do not rely on natural planning methods yet, as your body will not be in its regular rhythm for a bit. Of course, there is no shame in having babies close together, but if this is not your desire, have a plan.

Odor

Having some extra body odor after baby comes? This is common and due to all the hormone shifts you are experiencing. Speaking of odors, you may notice an odor "down there" as you recover. It may smell a bit off, but most of the time, it is normal—think an earthy smell. It can smell like a normal period or may be different and have more of a musty or stale odor. What you do not want is fishy or rotten odors. That would warrant a call to your healthcare provider.

Edema

Even if you did not swell in pregnancy, you may see some swollen feet, ankles, hands, and wrists early postpartum. Our bodies carry lots of extra fluid in pregnancy, and once our babies are born, our bodies have the task of getting rid of this fluid. I know it sounds counterintuitive, but drinking plenty of water will help you get rid of the fluid and swelling. Propping up your legs and feet can also help keep swelling controlled. Dry brushing is another technique that helps circulation and minimizes swelling.

Stretch Marks

Our bodies are master compensators. They do what we ask of them. When we are pregnant, our organs move out of the way, our ribs expand, and our breasts make colostrum. With these changes comes lots of stretching and growing. It is common to have stretch marks after pregnancy. In fact, 46.7 percent of women do.[9] So if you are standing side by side with another mom, one of you more than likely has some sort of stretch marks from pregnancy. It may be stretch marks on the belly, butt, or boobs (or any other place on your body). The good news is that stretch marks usually fade on their own over time. Those that remain are proof that we were a master of creating life!

More studies are needed on stretch-mark-reducing products, but I will give you the rundown on what the research shows. Cocoa butter was not any more effective than a placebo cream at reducing stretch marks; however, it did add elasticity and moisture to the skin. Olive oil had conflicting results, but some improvement was shown when used with massage. The same was true for bitter almond oil. Bio-Oil was proven effective on stretch marks on non-pregnant women, but research is still needed for pregnancy and postpartum.[10]

Studies found that the majority of the products used to reduce stretch marks were most effective with massage. If you choose to use a product, be sure to partner it with gentle massage so it has the greatest effect.

Postpartum Hair Loss

I have vivid memories of showering at four months postpartum and noticing more hair than normal rinsing out. It made me nervous, and I wondered, *How bad will this get? How far will it go?* Postpartum hair loss is normal and usually happens between two and four months postpartum. It is a bit deceptive, though. The real reason we lose so much hair postpartum is that our hair significantly decreases its normal shedding in pregnancy.[11] There is a pause, if you will. During postpartum, the scalp makes up for this time of not shedding and begins to get rid of all the excess hair.

This shedding can last for 6 to 24 weeks. There is some evidence that biotin, zinc, marine-derived protein (like specific collagens), or Omega-3 polyunsaturated fatty acids can reduce hair loss.[12] If you have really long hair, it may help to get a shorter cut since this can make the hair lighter and avoid more breakage. Remember, this too shall pass. It won't be long until your hair will balance out once again.

. . . .

As you care for your body, do not forget the massive changes it has already amazingly accomplished. Your uterus is a powerhouse muscle that sustained and birthed your baby beautifully. Your breasts have been preparing colostrum to nourish your baby as soon as they are born. Your brain and emotions have been resorting so you could bond well with your baby and make an easier journey into becoming mama. So, well done, my friend! Postpartum recovery is a journey you are well-suited to travel. Close your eyes, take a deep breath, and whisper, "Good job."

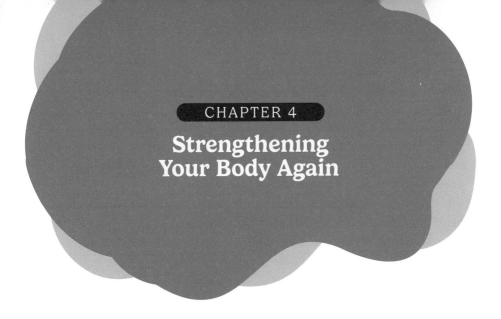

CHAPTER 4

Strengthening
Your Body Again

The term *bouncing back* causes different gut reactions. For some moms, this term makes them feel absolute rage because they understand how unrealistic this is. For others it makes them feel anxious that this may be an expectation when things already feel so overwhelming. And for others it feels like a challenge: a doable, accomplishable task. None are wrong.

Personally I would like to shelve this term. The idea of bouncing back comes with unattainable standards for most new mothers. Vulnerable moms (myself included!) often buy into the expectation that they should look a certain way or recover a certain way, and when reality does not meet expectations, these moms feel somehow less than all the other mothers. Shame begins to knock on our door, taunting us and telling us that if we admit to such a struggle, we will find we are alone. We believe the lie that recovery is easy for all other moms.

I much prefer the term *building back*. After all, this is what we're doing when we are recovering. We're healing strains or injuries, our organs are slowly moving back into place, our uteruses and bellies are slowly shrinking, all the while sustaining and caring for new humans. This should never be rushed, and the word *bouncing* does not fit this at all.

It would benefit us to vigilantly guard what we put in front of our eyes during this vulnerable postpartum time. The comparison game becomes too easy, especially when it comes to our changing bodies. Seeing an influencer post a photo of a fit six-week-postpartum body or a baby sleeping through the night at two weeks, without knowing what is truly going on behind the scenes, can be detrimental to the grace we give ourselves. And it is also important to remember that rushing fitness too early can actually hurt our recovery more than help it.

Physical Recovery

Like so many other new moms, my friend Maria was told not to exercise (or do much of anything) for six weeks after having her baby. Maria had always been a runner and looked forward to hitting the pavement once more. Six weeks postpartum came, and she laced up her Brooks running shoes. Off she went, only to find her pelvic floor was screaming at her and her bladder was not holding her urine. What happened?

Once we birth our babies, our bodies have gone through some of the biggest changes we will ever go through in a very short period of time. We are wonderful creations designed to accommodate pregnancy. When our babies are born, our backs probably have a bit of a sway to them, our abdominals have probably separated a bit to make room, our ribs have spread so everything could rearrange, and our ligaments have loosened to accommodate our growing baby and birth.

We are not just getting back in shape. We are healing, retraining our posture and alignment, and strengthening our pelvis again. Rushing through these details will cause further injury. But don't worry; we were made to adapt. As we introduce the right movements at the right time, we will heal appropriately, build strength, and come into proper alignment.

Though it is very important not to force ourselves to exercise for the first six weeks after having a baby, it also hinders our recovery to do absolutely nothing. Our bodies need to move. We need to stretch. I am not talking about doing high intensity interval training (HIIT) classes or weightlifting. That can be harmful when done too soon. But I am saying this is a process. To go from nothing to running at six weeks is not kind to our bodies.

NURSE'S TIP

Get fitted for new shoes. Often pregnancy changes our feet and arch support. When the feet are not properly supported, it affects the knees all the way to the pelvic floor. Care for your body by wearing supportive shoes!

It helps our physical bodies, our emotions, and our mental health to incorporate some form of movement into our day, whether that's taking our babies for a walk in their stroller or baby wearing and doing a short flexibility routine. You will never regret the effort you put into recovering and building strength back at the right time, in a kind way.

The six-week rule exists because studies show that women can safely begin activity at this point no matter their delivery outcomes. But the truth is that some women are ready to start activity several weeks prior.[1] Multiple factors come into play with this, though, such as fitness levels before delivery, the degree of tear or episiotomy, and C-section birth. Fitness progress is built, not miraculously gifted to us by a healthcare provider.

Though we know new moms deal with physical exhaustion and interrupted sleep, we also know prolonged sedentary lifestyles lead to more exhaustion, less mental acuity, and depression. For moms who are already at risk for emotional upheaval and postpartum depression, this is bad news. Leaving out physical movement makes us *more* tired than incorporating it into our lives.[2] Many research studies tell us that regular exercise needs to be a priority in the postpartum period for reducing stress and depression.[3]

It would benefit new mothers to have an individualized plan for getting back to fitness that considers their fitness history and birth stories. But for many of us, a personal trainer is simply out of the question. It is vital to assess yourself when deciding what you are ready for. You know yourself better than anyone. If at three weeks postpartum you feel ready to move, go for it; but start slow and low according to the guidelines I'm going to give you. Meaning, even if you did boxing HIIT classes up until delivery, let's not start with that.

I will always advise you to check with your healthcare provider before starting any exercises. I think that is wisdom. I have not had the privilege of taking care of you personally or knowing all of your health history. But after working with postpartum mothers, a personal trainer, and my pelvic floor physical therapists, I have designed the 5 Kind Movements for the postpartum body.[4] These are gentle movements specifically for the recovering postpartum body that ease you into flexibility and strength regardless of prior training. They will help you get back into your regular fitness routines as well. More on those in a bit.

Rest

Many midwives ascribe to the 5-5-5 Rule when it comes to rest. Have you heard of this before? Basically, the first 15 days after birth look something like this:

- 5 days *in* the bed: laying down, resting as much as possible.
- 5 days *on* the bed: sitting up in the bed, resting when needed.
- 5 days *near* the bed: still in the bedroom, maybe up in a rocking chair, but hanging out close to the bed.

Emphasize resting for the first two weeks after birth, and never rush. This allows you time to get to know your baby, to bond with them, and learn their cues. It helps you establish good breastfeeding. It also puts you in the right mindset to go slow and recover gently.

The 5-5-5 Rule is not meant to restrict a mom who needs to move. Mothers with other children or who do not have a supportive partner may find this sort of rest to be an impossible task. This rule was not meant to put another burden on your shoulders. It is simply there to give you the permission to rest if you are able. You know yourself and your situation best. If you need to move around, do so while paying attention to your body's signals to rest.

I don't recommend doing any exercise for the first two weeks after birth. This time should be focused on perineal care and taking care of your basic needs and the needs of your baby. While some women want to begin slow movement after two weeks, some will not feel ready for six weeks. That's okay! We are all different.

NURSE'S TIP

When resting, be sure to spend time horizontally, not just sitting up. Laying flat will keep pressure off of a healing pelvic floor.

In getting back to physical activity, being realistic with your goals is a big deal. Before pregnancy, if you plan to run a 5K with no training or prep work, you may make it to the finish line, but you're liable to not lift a finger again for weeks. Your body will be sore and uncomfortable because it wasn't trained for such a task. This doesn't benefit us. How much more should we be aware of the need to give ourselves time to build our strength and abilities after the changes of birth? Goals should be simple and achievable.

Showing up is another big deal. Progress is progress, no matter how small. When it's time, if you have a plan to work in ten minutes of activity three days a week, do it. Do what it takes to get it in. You may have to wear your baby in a carrier to accomplish it or sit them in their bouncy seat where they can see you, but each day you show up is a chapter in the story of your health. Be there for yourself.

QUESTION:
Should I do Kegels?

ANSWER: Rachel Moran, pelvic floor physical therapist states, "Kegels can be beneficial for some people, but not everyone. It is most important that we teach the pelvic floor to function in a system with our gluteal and abdominal muscles. Focusing on strengthening our bigger muscles groups, like the core and glutes, can help strengthen the pelvic floor more than anything. And remember, relaxing everything is just as important as tightening."[5]

Kegels

Once upon a time, the extent of our pelvic floor recovery advice was to do Kegels, which are a great exercise for what they are. They are used to tighten the pelvic floor. But our goal is not necessarily a tight pelvic floor; our goal is a strong pelvic floor. We want it to be able to do its job of holding organs and providing continence.

Runners, athletes, and yogis often have a very tight pelvic floor. These women may be in great shape and yet find a C-section birth necessary because their pelvic floor did not yield to their baby's head. Working with a pelvic floor physical therapist can help women achieve a supple pelvic floor before birth and after. The therapist will give exercises that can help too!

Many women are eager to begin Kegels after giving birth, and for that reason I am including instructions on how to do a proper Kegel. But we know through research and practice that incorporating specialized movements like lunges, squats, and bridges builds strength and is more effective to building pelvic floor health than doing Kegels alone.[6] Healthcare professionals (myself, pelvic floor physical therapists, and others) also know that many women think they are doing a correct Kegel but are not. If you are only going to choose one or the other, I recommend the Five Kind Movements over Kegels alone.

To do a Kegel properly, lie on your back, side, or belly, whichever feels best. You can also lie flat on your back with your feet rested against a wall. No distractions are best when first learning to do Kegels. First, take a couple of deep breaths to connect with your body. Now begin by taking a deep inhale (draw your breath slowly in), and then as you slowly exhale, imagine picking up a blueberry with your vagina. Draw up and in like you are lifting that blueberry. Your butt should be relaxed. When it is time to inhale again, put the blueberry back down.

Relaxing your pelvic floor is just as important as tightening it. Think of the pelvic floor like another muscle in the body. If I were to decide to strengthen my biceps by doing 100 curls a day, they would definitely get stronger. But if I never lengthened and stretched the muscle, it would lose flexibility and the ability to recover, and it would be more prone to injury. The pelvic floor is the same. Take time to put the blueberry back down. You may notice you can feel the Kegel better in certain positions. When I first started Kegels, I felt it best when lying on my stomach. This helped me learn how to do it, so I could use other positions.

Emily Gilmore, pelvic floor physical therapist and owner of Thrive Physical Therapy and Wellness, states, "The pelvic floor stretches two to three times its normal resting length for birth. To put this in perspective, the bicep can only stretch around one times its length." In other words, the pelvic floor stretches 250 percent of its resting length.[7] What a stretch! It's no wonder the goal of pelvic floor work in the fourth trimester is rebuilding strength.

When I birthed my babies, my healthcare provider did not discuss the need for pelvic floor health, and I had no idea therapy was an option. It was only when my third baby was six years old that I noticed signs of pelvic floor dysfunction. For me, it was spotting when exercising. For others, it's leaking pee when working out or feeling heavy in the vagina with any physical activity. Some professionals may tell you, "It's normal" or ,"It just happens after having babies." But by this point, I knew better, and I asked my OB for a referral to a pelvic floor physical therapist. (Not all states require physician referrals for physical therapy, but mine currently does.)

As I worked with her, things began to improve. My body and pelvic floor needed some help to do their job well. But the moral of the story is that it is not too late to get some help. Whether you had your baby two months ago or ten years ago, you don't have to suffer through symptoms. There is hope.

Though pelvic floor health has long been an area of focus in France, here in the US, we are just beginning to catch on. Thankfully, we are learning fast and many insurance companies are now covering a pelvic floor physical therapist in the fourth trimester. Though it is not a standard of postpartum care yet (but I believe it soon will be), I highly recommend scheduling a physical therapy appointment between six and eight weeks postpartum if you are able. A skilled pelvic floor physical therapist will be able to assess exactly where you need work and create a plan for your pelvic floor to fully recover.

Breathe First

Becoming aware of our breath and being able to breathe during movement is a sign that you are ready to move forward with some physical activity. If you find that you are holding your breath during movement, you are not getting the focused benefits of the exercise you are doing. Slow down. Focus on the breath again. Get this right before moving forward.

To practice breathing mindfully, lie flat on your back with your feet on the floor and knees toward the ceiling. Place your right hand on your stomach and left hand on your heart. Inhale deeply through your nose while aiming to lift your stomach and chest at the same time. You'll know you're doing this correctly when both hands rise simultaneously. Exhale through your nose. Both hands should lower at the same time. This practice helps build a good foundation for breath work, decreases unnecessary pelvic tilt, and helps protect your form when you begin adding movement to your regimen.

QUESTION:
Am I ready for exercise?

ANSWER: You are usually ready to begin exercising when you can go for a ten-minute walk while controlling the breaths you take, without seeing an increase in bleeding or starting to bleed again if your bleeding has already stopped.

Walk Second

Walking is incredibly underrated. It has numerous benefits like increasing your range of motion, lengthening your psoas muscle, aiding with flexibility, adding balance, and building your skeletal muscular system.[8] (The psoas are long muscles that connect your core to your lower body. They are responsible for motion and flexion between many body parts, especially the spine and hips.[9]) Building the skeletal muscular system is especially important for women at risk for osteopenia (low bone density), like older moms and vegans. For the first three to four weeks postpartum, keep a walk to under 15 minutes. After four weeks postpartum, choosing to walk for ten minutes three times per day, three days a week protects bone density and also helps lead to emotional peace.

When you feel you are ready to move, do yourself a favor and go for a short, ten-minute walk. How did it feel? If it felt uncomfortable or downright painful, wait another week and try again. If you are tolerating ten-minute walks without seeing an increase in vaginal bleeding, and you can control your breath while walking, you are ready to try the Five Kind Movements.

The Five Kind Movements

I created the Five Kind Movements specifically for the postpartum body. These moves are made to connect you back to your body while gently strengthening and adding a bit of flexibility. They will ease you back into physical activity the right way, so you can have an easier time getting back to doing what you love (video version available at MamaDidIt.com).

When you're ready to add movement to your life (not before the first two weeks postpartum), you have practiced your breath work, and you can take a walk according to the mentioned guidelines, I recommend doing this set once through for three to five days per week to start. It will take around 15 minutes to complete. Don't rush through the movements. The goal is to connect to your body again, connect with your core muscles, and begin to add movement and strength back to your life.

Always check in with your breath. If you are going through the Five Kind Movements and you can't do them without holding your breath, go back to simple breathing techniques and ten-minute walks. Try the Movements again a week or two later.

You'll notice that a couple of these movements incorporate a pelvic floor contraction (Kegel). This is because of the research we looked at earlier. Incorporating a pelvic floor contraction with a specialized movement is more effective at strengthening the pelvic floor than Kegels alone.

Equipment needed: a playground ball, 9-inch physio ball, Stoked ball, or a pillow

MOVEMENT 1: MINI FLOW

Why you need it: Improves strength and flexibility in the back, glutes, hamstrings, arms, shoulders, wrists, and pelvis. Wakes up the body. Engages pelvic floor muscles and can help avoid pelvic dysfunction.

How to do it:

1. From a standing position, take a deep breath and inhale with arms up overhead. Slowly swan dive forward (reach your fingertips towards your toes) and put your hands on the ground in front of you. It's okay to bend your knees so you can reach the floor.

2. Walk your hands out until you are in a plank position. If you need to modify by placing a knee or two on the floor to get to a plank, feel free. Push through the palms of your hands and push your butt into the air. Drop your heels towards the floor. You should feel a stretch in your calf muscles. Hold for five seconds while you breathe. This is a downward dog position.

3. Roll your body forward, and slowly lower yourself back towards plank position, but continue all the way to the floor. With tummy resting on the floor, flatten the front of your feet to the ground, and lift the chest up while resting on your elbows to a modified cobra pose. Hold for five seconds while breathing.

4. From modified cobra, push up on your hands to plank position and repeat the flow by moving back into downward dog. Repeat.

How many times: Twice

When the flow is complete, come down to all fours, and move on to Movement 2.

MOVEMENT 2: DIAPHRAGMATIC BREATHING IN QUADRUPED

Why you need it: Lowers cortisol, provides mind-body connection, makes core exercises more effective, and improves core muscle stability.

How to do it:

1. Get on all fours. Find your straight back. Do not round or arch your back. Use a mirror if you need to.
2. As you inhale, fill the belly up with breath. Your ribs should expand, and your belly should get bigger.
3. Exhale and pull the belly in toward your spine while keeping the back straight. Contract the pelvic floor on the exhale if you can.
4. Repeat.

How many times: 10 times

MOVEMENT 3: OPEN BOOK

Why you need it: Stretches the chest, shoulders, and upper back, helps with spinal mobility, improves neck discomfort, helps with proper postural alignment. It is especially needed for mothers who are holding babies or breastfeeding often.

How to do it:

1. Lie on your side with both hands extended out in front of you, palms of the hands together. You can place a pillow behind your head and between your knees for extra support if needed.
2. Squeeze your knees together firmly. Slowly raise your top hand toward the ceiling and extend it behind you, opening up your back and chest until your hand rests on the floor. If you cannot go all the way to the floor, it's okay. Go as far as you can comfortably go. Your hips should stay still. Be sure to breathe.

3. Bring the arm slowly back over your body until it is resting once again in the start position. Repeat.

How many times: 6 on each side

MOVEMENT 4: HEEL SLIDES

Why you need it: Strengthens the core, stabilizes the pelvis, strengthens the leg muscles.

How to do it:

1. Lay flat on your back with feet planted on the floor and knees pointed at the ceiling. Drop your belly button toward your spine and make sure your lower back stays plastered to the floor.

2. Push your heel along the floor slowly until the leg is straight. As you push the leg out, slowly inhale.

3. As you pull the leg back to you, think of drawing it in with your lower abdominal muscles. Exhale as you bring it back in. Repeat with the opposite side.

How many times: 6 on each leg

MOVEMENT 5: BRIDGES WITH KEGELS

Why you need it: Releases your low back, stabilizes your core, strengthens your butt and hamstrings, strengthens your pelvic floor.

How to do it:

1. Lay on your back with your knees pointed toward the ceiling and feet planted on the floor. Do not let your knees cave in or fall outward. Keep the legs stable.

2. Place a ball or pillow between the knees for stability. Shimmy your hands from side to side and see if you can graze your heels with your fingertips. If you can, you are in the right position.

3. Lift your butt to a glute engaged position, not a hyperextended position. We are not trying to thrust at the ceiling. As you lift, gently squeeze the ball and contract the pelvic floor (Kegel) if you can. Keep your core engaged. Exhale while you lift.

4. Squeeze your booty at the top for three seconds. Relax the Kegel and inhale as you lower back down.

How many times: 10

Your goals with the Five Kind Movements are to move through all five, as written, with proper form and good breath work (inhaling on the easy part of the exercise and exhaling on the exertion part). Once this begins to feel natural, move through the Five Kind Movements twice on your work-out days. Once this begins to feel natural, and you can still maintain proper form and breath work, move through them three times. By the time you can do three sets of these movements several days per week, you are ready to move on to other workouts as you feel able.

Keep a long-term focus when you are working on building back. You will not drop weight fast or gain loads of muscle overnight, but that's not the goal. Our goal is healing well, increasing our strength and flexibility, connecting with our body and core again, and building back energy and health in a kind way. You'll find that after just a few weeks, you're feeling stronger, a bit more confident, and in a better headspace than before you started.

Diastasis Recti

Women in the last several years have become much more aware of the term *diastasis recti*. This is thanks to focus and attention from birth workers and personal trainers. Diastasis recti is a separation of the rectus abdominis muscles (the same area as the six-pack). It can happen as our wombs grow and need more room for our babies. There is no sure-fire way to prevent this, but flexibility routines give our bodies more room to give in other ways, and choosing not to wear a bra, when possible, can give our ribs room to move and our uterus more room to go up than out.[10] It's important to know that this is a normal adaptation of our body when pregnant. It does not mean you did something wrong! The good news is that over 60 percent of diastasis recti cases resolve on their own in the fourth trimester.[11]

Therapeutic exercise is beneficial for fixing diastasis recti that doesn't resolve on its own. It's best to do these exercises under the supervision of a pelvic floor physical therapist. Though belly binders have shown some benefits for helping to reconnect the abdominal muscles after diastasis recti, they are not as effective as safe exercise. The Five Kind Movements are safe to do with diastasis recti and may help reconnection of these tissues. Avoid exercises that involve extended planking times or moves with upper body twisting, like Russian twists. This can put too much pressure on the area and hinder it from reconnecting.

Belly Wrapping and Belly Binding

If you do a deep dive on postpartum belly binding, you will find a rich history of all different kinds of wrapping and techniques. This practice goes back for centuries. Most women may benefit from belly binding, but there are a few things to consider.

Belly binding or wrapping may be helpful, but studies also tell us that wearing binders can increase intraabdominal pressure.[12] This means binding too tightly can put more strain on an already struggling or injured pelvic floor. We certainly do not want to impede recovery or healing here! If you are seeing a pelvic floor physical therapist, they can help you decide whether these binders are right for you. Here are a few questions to ask yourself to determine if you need one:

- Have you had a C-section? Most C-section moms need the support of a belly binder.

- Do you feel like you need one? If you feel you would benefit from one, you probably would.

- Do you feel like your "guts are hanging out" when you try to
  walk? Use a belly binder for support.

To wrap appropriately, hold the belly binder behind your back with one
side in each hand. Pull one side tightly around your abdomen. Pull the
other side tightly around as well and Velcro in place. Some women bind
over the hips and some above them. Do what feels best to you, and if your
wrap comes with instructions, use them. It should feel like gentle but firm
support. A belly binder should never be so tight that it hinders taking a
deep breath. At times it is helpful to let a support person wrap it for you,
or to lie down on your back with the belly binder behind you. This helps it
stay in place as you wrap and Velcro.

· · · · · · · · · · · ·

As you rest, recover, and begin to build back, remember, this is not a
race. It is a slow climb up the mountain of recovery. But you will find that
as you listen to your body and build back well, you can feel more whole
than you have ever felt before.

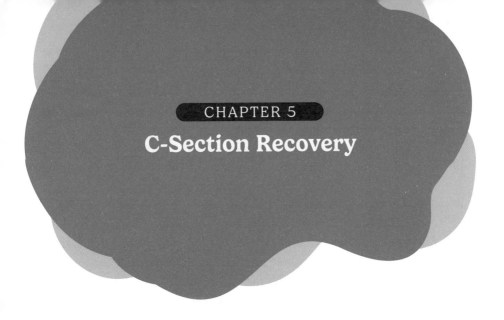

CHAPTER 5

C-Section Recovery

S arah had been pushing for four hours. As she fell back in exhaustion between contractions, her thoughts slipped to the early hours of the morning. She had felt so certain, so sure, of how this day would go. Early labor would be managed at home. She would do the proper positions and movements to give her baby the best advantage for easing through the birth canal.

What is happening? What did I do wrong? she pondered. She struggled with feeling completely helpless as her birth story unfolded in a way she had never expected.

She is not alone. You are not alone.

Currently, over 30 percent of women in America have cesarean sections.[1] Many are unplanned. The stories of how they end up having a cesarean section versus having a vaginal birth vary tremendously. Whether the mom was diagnosed with failure to progress, was too exhausted to push, had an umbilical cord wrapped around the baby causing a low heart rate, baby was simply not handling the contractions well, or the mom's blood pressure was too high, the results are the same—cesarean birth.

C-sections are wonderful when needed. They allow medical staff to help a struggling baby or mother to give birth in as little as two minutes if need be. This surgery has saved many lives and helped achieve the outcome that we all desire, a healthy mother and baby.

Of course, any type of surgery comes with recovery and possible complications. C-section moms face a longer and harder physical recovery as well as possibly needing transitional care for their newborns. They may also have failed expectations of their birth story and need to mourn this loss.

There are also mothers who planned for this birth story and scheduled a C-section. They knew what to expect, and they did the research and prepared accordingly. Typically, these mothers do not experience the grief that unplanned cesarean sections can bring.

A mother who didn't count on a C-section may experience feelings of powerlessness, disappointment, and grief. I have seen patients experience post-traumatic stress disorder (PTSD) when their birth did not go as planned. These feelings are real and valid and can contribute to postpartum depression and postpartum anxiety. "It's not supposed to be this way," is a true expression of grief and dashed hopes.

As I have sat across from many a new mother who shared tears with me over her C-section birth story, one theme was prevalent. She felt like less of a woman for not having a vaginal birth. I thought, *How could this be?* When she would ask if I had experienced a C-section, and I replied that I had not, I could see shame wash over her face. She was telling herself a story that somehow, she was less of a woman and a mother for having had this type of birth.

I simply could not believe it. I have seen so many new mothers forced to let go of expectations they had counted on—planned, ideal births. Maybe their baby had to spend some time in the NICU. Maybe they pushed for hours as the mother did at the beginning of this chapter only to have a C-section. And they would grieve, somehow believing they were less for it.

Mama, listen to me here. You had your body ripped open to deliver your baby. Yes, grieve. Yes, process those feelings. But never forget that you, just like Jesus, had your side split open for your children (John 19:34). You laid down your life, your expectations, your plans, your choices, and your hopes, to get your baby here safely. That is superhero status! You are no less of a mother because you had a C-section.

The Big Things After a C-Section

If you have a C-Section you have come out of childbirth not only with a newborn to care for, but also with a body recovering from surgery. It's easy to forget that you are recovering from major abdominal surgery. Many moms are so focused on caring for their babies that they forget to care for themselves. Isn't this the most motherhood thing ever?

Bleeding

The bleeding you have after a C-section is similar to a vaginal delivery. The good news is that C-section moms tend to only bleed for two to three weeks, as opposed to four to six. They also don't usually bleed as heavily. Vaginal bleeding after birth, you may recall, is called lochia; it is not the same as a period. This bleeding comes from a combination of tissue, blood, and mucous that your womb sheds after giving birth.

NURSE'S TIP

Do not use ointments like Neosporin on C-section incisions. These ointments can dissolve the glue used in surgery and reopen the incision.

Gas Pain

A fellow nurse came to me one shift and said, "I've done everything I can for this patient's pain, and she is still hurting so bad. I don't know what to do." I agreed to go talk to the patient. I asked her a few questions, and when she said, "I'm hurting so bad in my shoulder." I knew exactly what to do.

I said, "I think you are having gas pain."

She looked at me quite aggravated and stated matter-of-factly, "This *is not* gas pain."

I replied, "Okay. But you've tried everything else. Why not just try some Gas-X and see if it happens to work?"

She reluctantly agreed. Thirty minutes later I saw her walking in the hall and asked how she felt. She excitedly said, "I can't believe that was gas pain!" I laughed and told her I was glad she felt better.

Gas pain after a C-section often is not felt like normal gas pain. It tends to radiate to the shoulder and can feel sharp and very painful. Shoulder pain after surgery usually points to trapped gas. Walking around, avoiding straws, limiting carbonated drinks, and taking some gas reliever should do the trick!

Incisional Pain

Incisional pain usually feels like burning, stinging, or a hot iron. Using an ice pack on your incision, especially for the first couple of days, can relieve pain. Don't be a hero here! (You already are one.) Take your pain medicine when you need it. You will definitely need it in the hospital, but you will also probably need it off and on for a few days once you get home. Incisional pain should get better each day.

Many nursing moms feel concerned about pain medication passing to their baby through their breast milk. Controlled substances, like narcotics, do pass through breast milk, but when pain is not effectively controlled, it can cause our milk supply not to let down for our baby to nurse. Most professionals advise mom to nurse first, then take her pain medication. This gives your body time to break down the medicine, so your baby gets minimal amounts that doesn't affect them.

Using the Bathroom

It may be tough to feel when you need to pee the first few days after surgery. Moms will often tell me their incision hurts, but after palpating, I find their bladder is distended. Once they pee, the pain goes away. For this reason, try to urinate every few hours even if you don't feel like you need to go.

It's best to take a laxative and stool softener combination (like Senokot), as directed, after a C-section delivery. The bowels can be sluggish after surgery. Other factors like narcotic pain medications can also cause constipation. Taking a laxative and stool softener combo can keep things moving until you are regular again.

Afterbirth Pain

C-section moms, just like vaginal delivery moms, will have afterbirth pains (or after pains). These are cramps that can feel intense the first couple days after birth. Though it doesn't feel like it, they are doing your body a favor. It is the uterus clamping down to prevent too much bleeding. These afterbirth pains are also helping your uterus return to prepregnancy size. Though this pain feels more intense after each baby we birth, the cramps themselves get better with each passing day. A heating pad, reusable hot pack, or over-the-counter ibuprofen can bring relief.

QUESTION:
When can I drive after a C-section?

ANSWER: Never drive if you are still taking narcotic medications. Once off the medication, try this test first: Kick your tire. If it hurts, you are not ready to drive. If it does not, go for it. If you experienced pain, you may be unable to brake quickly, which can cause a crash. Most moms can drive two weeks after surgery.

Coughing and Laughing

"Stop making me laugh!" one of my moms told her husband as he joked around with her the day after her surgery. Pain when coughing and laughing can cause extra discomfort in a C-section mama. It causes movement in the belly and can pull on the C-section incision. To help prevent this, grab a pillow and hold it firmly over your lower tummy. This helps to brace your healing incision and will keep you from jarring your incision as much.

Incisional Care

Have you seen the silicone scar patches or the C-Panties made especially for C-section moms? Though these brands are new to the postpartum market, silicone gel sheeting has been used for more than 30 years as a first line of defense in scar therapy.[2] These products can be very helpful for reducing the appearance of your C-section scar, but they should not be used until your incision has completely closed and healed, and no drainage or scabbing is present.

You may see some drainage from the incision as it heals. This can be clear or pink-tinged, and it's a normal part of healing. In the meantime, follow your doctor's instructions for incision care. If you have staples, you will have them taken out around one week postpartum. If you have stitches covered with Steri-Strips, take the strips off one week postpartum (unless your doctor says otherwise). The main thing with incision care is keeping it clean and dry. When you shower, gently clean with soapy water, rinse off, and pat to towel dry. If your belly consistently covers your incision, keeping it overly moist, you can occasionally place a maxi pad over the area to help keep it dry as it heals.

Incisional Numbness

Though physicians take care to prevent it, sometimes an incision in surgery can sever a nerve in the area. This can lead to numbness of the incision in whole or in part. Sometimes this numbness can reverse, but sometimes it is permanent. Some moms appreciate this numbness because it helps with pain control. Others find it annoying. Either way, incisional numbness becomes much like a stretch mark. It's proof that we created life!

Sex

Though I cover sex extensively in chapter 18, I want to touch on it here. Often C-section parents have not been told why they should not have sex too early after surgery. The same six-week rule of no sex applies to C-sections just as it does vaginal births. Even though your baby did not come through your birth canal, your placenta still left a large wound in your uterus. Having sex too early can introduce infection into your womb. Plus, if you were in labor and your cervix dilated, it needs around six weeks to close up completely. It is best to wait the full six weeks before having sex again.

Bathing and Swimming

Most healthcare providers agree that it is best to avoid taking a bath or swimming until vaginal bleeding has stopped completely after a vaginal or C-section birth. It's also a good idea to wait until your C-section incision has zero drainage and your Steri-Strips or staples have been removed before swimming. Swimming too early can introduce infection to a healing uterus and incision.

The good news is that vaginal discharge tends to stop a couple of weeks sooner with a C-section than with a vaginal birth. A C-section mama may be able to return to a pool or bath a bit quicker than a vaginal birth mama thanks to this. With a cesarean section, it's usually safe to submerge in water at four weeks if the guidelines mentioned have been met.

Helpful Tips After a C-Section

Getting Up and Down

Once you are up, you are usually good, and once you are down, you are usually good. (Reminds me of an old Sunday School song.) It is the in-between that is hard. If you have a two-level home, plan to stay on one level as much as you can. Taking the stairs is okay, but it can be tiring and uncomfortable after a C-section.

Some Tips for Getting Up

- Get up like a mermaid. Keep your feet, ankles, and knees together and move both legs as one. This takes the strain off your tummy.

- Push up out of bed with your arms instead of using your stomach muscles to pull you up.

- Once you are sitting up, intentionally use your leg muscles to push your body up. This will also keep the strain off your incision and stomach muscles.

- Brace your stomach with a pillow for extra support while you stand up, if needed.

Use a Rolling Cart

Make it easier for yourself by preparing a rolling cart. Stock your cart with frequently used supplies like a water bottle, snacks, meds, hair ties, a diaper-changing station, breastfeeding supplies, and changes of clothes for your baby. Also add any creams, lanolin, or tinctures you use often. Having this ready to roll not only keeps everything in arm's reach, but also allows you to easily move the cart to another room if you need to change your location.

QUESTION:
Do I need pelvic floor physical therapy after a C-section?

ANSWER: Emily Gilmore, pelvic floor physical therapist, states, "Oftentimes C-section moms don't think they need rehab or believe they are exempt from common postpartum problems. The opposite is true. These moms typically benefit from core strengthening, scar mobilization, postural retraining, as well as pelvic floor intervention. We recommend an appointment between six to eight weeks postpartum."[3]

Touch Therapy

"Do you want to see your incision?" I have often asked my C-section mamas as I take their bandage off for them. Some are interested and others give me a firm, "No way!" The no's most often come from the moms who did not plan for a C-section. They may be feeling disconnected from their bodies or dealing with disappointment and grief.

Incorporating some touch therapy can help you begin to tell your body and brain that "It's okay. I'm okay." If you completely avoid the incisional area, as the nerves begin to reintegrate and heal, anything that comes near your incision, like underwear and pants, can feel painful. You can help your nerves reintegrate by introducing touch through this process. Using your hand, gently touch and stroke your upper abdomen. Move to the sides of your abdomen. No need to touch the incision. When you feel ready, move to your belly button area. Using touch therapy helps you reconnect your body to your brain.

Belly Wrapping and Belly Binding

Belly binding is always encouraged after a C-section. Studies have found that using a belly binder after a C-section helps with pain, increases a mom's ability to get out of bed and walk around, and helps her feel better supported in recovery.[4]

I have found that belly binders with Velcro are the easiest to work with. Many C-section moms bind over their hips and tummy because it helps their incision area feel protected. Some moms wrap standing up while looking in the mirror and some lay the wrap on their bed, lay down on it, and wrap their stomachs this way. Do what feels best to you. Wrap tightly enough for your stomach to feel supported, but not so tightly that you can't take a deep breath. Asking a support person to wrap it for you can help.

· · · · · · · · · · · ·

Don't forget, Mama, a C-section is major abdominal surgery. You not only are recovering from birth and caring for a newborn, but you are also recovering from surgery. You may have good days and you may have rough days. This is to be expected. Give yourself lots of grace and take each day one step at a time. A rough day does not mean you are not getting better. It probably means you need to rest a bit more.

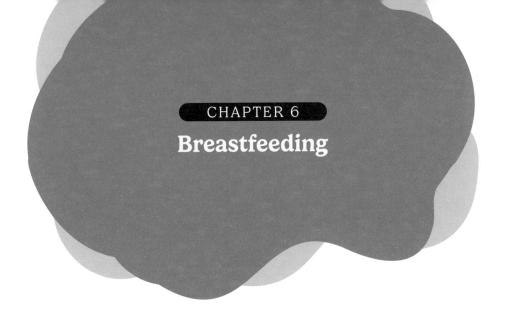

CHAPTER 6

Breastfeeding

Breastfeeding is natural, but that does not mean it will be easy. Many moms enter the breastfeeding process with the expectation that things are going to be perfect. But this is a natural process that may take time and practice to get the hang of.

I have birthed three children, and with each of them, the breastfeeding experience was totally different. With my first, I had more discomfort than I expected. This gave me a whole new empathy for my own patients! A professional offered me a nipple shield, a silicone shield that covers the nipple, and I gladly accepted. But I wish I had been told that a nipple shield, when used long-term, can decrease your milk supply and make it hard for your baby to latch without it. The nipple should also be centered in the shield, and the shield rolled inside out a bit before popping it onto the nipple. These are all instructions that I didn't receive! My nipple shield and I became one for the next eight months. That is, until my milk supply had tanked so much that it didn't make sense for me to nurse anymore.

If it comes down to giving up breastfeeding or using a nipple shield, use the shield. When you are ready to step away from the shield, try nursing for a few minutes with it, then take it away and see if your baby can latch on without it. It may take several days of being consistent with this process, but it usually works to wean a baby off the shield.

I'm going to share with you what I wish I had known: Nursing is usually uncomfortable when you have never done it before. It is normal for your nipples to hurt the first few seconds after your baby latches on. After that, though, you should not have pain. Your baby's tug should be strong and firm, but you adapt to this. You should not be in tears during your entire nursing session! This can point to a latch issue that needs to be worked on.

My second baby was a whole other story. I could not get the hang of nursing her without my nipples becoming cracked and bleeding. I ended up pumping and feeding her from a bottle for several months before giving up and putting her on formula. I later learned that she probably had a tongue tie, and this was the source of all our issues. Clicking and smacking while feeding can be signs of a baby's inability to get a deep enough latch due to a tongue tie. If you suspect a tongue tie, ask a lactation consultant or your pediatrician to check for it.

And then there was my third. Though he tried to tuck his bottom lip under while nursing (which can cause breastfeeding discomfort), nursing with him was how I had initially expected it to go with all my babies. He breastfed well from the start. His latch was right, and my milk supply was adequate. Weaning was the only question mark I had with him. After turning to breastfeeding blogs and Google searches, I learned that he would wean when ready.

Nope. No natural weaning for us. After the first couple of years of nursing him, I took a trip away and simply had to quit cold turkey. Here's the lesson I learned through this experience: What works for some mothers won't always work for *all* mothers.

What You Should Know

So what should you expect while breastfeeding? Here's what I have learned after caring for thousands of breastfeeding mamas. There are a few tried and true guidelines for "normal," but lots of little issues can come up along the way. We will look at several of those issues and how to resolve them.

First, you should expect exclusively breastfed babies to nurse every 2 to 3 hours until you choose to introduce formula or solid foods. This equals a total of 8-12 feedings every 24 hours (this includes night feedings). Most babies will nurse around 20 minutes per breast. But there is no need to stop a baby from nursing off one breast if they are not done in 20 minutes. Think of the first breast as the main meal, and the second breast as dessert. Always rotate which breast you start on each time you nurse to help equal out milk supply.

Time your baby's feed time from the time they start nursing, not the time they finish. Give them a burp between breasts, but also be aware that they may not burp. Breastfed babies get very little air while nursing. The American Academy of Pediatrics recommends exclusively breastfeeding for at least the first six months of your baby's life.[1]

NORMAL BREASTFEEDING PATTERNS

- Babies nurse every 2-3 hours
- Babies feed 8-12 times every 24 hours
- Babies nurse around 20 minutes per side
- Rotate the side you start on with each feeding
- There will be times your baby wants to nurse more frequently. This is called *cluster feeding* and indicates a growth spurt. This usually lasts 2-3 days.

When Will My Milk Come In?

During pregnancy, our breasts are making colostrum for our babies. This is waiting and ready for whenever birth comes. There is not much volume to colostrum, but it's nutrition packed and is even considered our baby's first immunization because of its infection-fighting ability. Colostrum (except in rare circumstances) is enough for our babies as long as they are latching well and often. For a first-time mama, mature breast milk comes in around day three to five. Moms who have C-sections may see a breast-milk delay by one day or so more. A mama who has nursed before may see her mature milk come in within as little as 36 hours after birth.

Milk let-down is different than your milk coming in. Milk coming in refers to the first time your colostrum transitions to mature breast milk. Milk let-down is when your milk "drops" into your breast for your baby at each feeding. This may be accompanied by an emotional low or tears thanks to hormone shifts. It may also feel tingly, like pins and needles, warm, heavy, or with a burning sensation.

Scheduling Feedings

When you hear that babies need to eat every two to three hours, it's good to know that this is a guideline. Rarely will you ever be exactly at hour two or three. Go by your baby's cues to know when it is time to feed. This may be two hours, or it could be one hour if they are in a growth spurt.

Jess was a patient of mine who had given birth to her baby the night before. She was rightfully exhausted and asked the nurse to take her little one to the nursery for three hours so she could sleep. At hour one, her baby began to show hunger cues (putting her hands to her mouth, smacking, and turning her head to find a breast). Her nurse attempted to take the baby back, but mom refused. She had been educated by a social media graphic that her baby should not be hungry yet. The nurse, wanting to keep the patient happy, took the baby back to the nursery for another hour. By this point, the baby was restless and crying (a late hunger sign). She took her back to her mother and once again, she said she could not be hungry yet. It took a nursing supervisor to properly reeducate the mother that her baby was indeed hungry, and it was not wise to go by arbitrary time frames.

HOW MUCH BREASTMILK DO BABIES NEED?

Baby's Tummy Size:

- Marble: Days 1-3
- Walnut: Day 3 to 2 weeks
- Ping Pong Ball: 2 weeks to 4 weeks

Many new moms worry if their baby is getting enough. It helps to remember that a baby's tummy is small.

Can My Baby Skip a Feeding at Night?

It's safe to say that your baby can skip a nighttime feeding if they are feeding at least 8-12 times in 24 hours. In other words, if skipping a night feeding does not drop them to seven feedings in 24 hours, you're good to take advantage of the extra sleep. It's also important to note that you should be confident that nursing is going well and that your milk supply is adequate before skipping feedings. Another question to ask is, "Is my baby gaining weight?" If you can answer yes to weight gain, good milk supply, and enough feedings, it's okay to let your baby sleep through a feeding at night if they so desire. If you ever have questions about nursing your baby, check with your healthcare provider.

> ## NURSE'S TIP
> ....
> The safest place to nurse your baby at night is in
> the bed with you. Push big pillows and blankets
> away, so if your baby falls asleep, they are safe
> in the bed with you until one of you wakes.

Proper Positioning

When I chatted with Jordan Clarke, lactation consultant (IBCLC) and founder of Birmingham Breastfeeding, I asked for her best positioning tips for new mothers. Here is what she had to say.

- Lie back a bit. Moms tend to feel the need to lean over and support their baby in their own strength. This leads to tension and discomfort as well as a poor latch. Rather than sitting up at a 90-degree angle or slumping toward your baby, recline back some, relax, and bring your baby to you. The slight recline encourages gravity to do the work of keeping the baby close to you, giving you the freedom to relax.

- Use a lumbar pillow. This will help support your lower back while you lean back and relax your shoulders.

- Position your baby tummy to tummy. This keeps a baby as close to their mom as possible. I love to think about how we eat at a table—our whole body is facing the table. The same holds true for our babies. Their whole body needs to be aligned facing their mom. When we combine reclining and relaxing our bodies with our baby turned completely toward us, it results in a more vigorous feeder. There is also the bonus of letting gravity work in our favor. (For C-section moms who feel uncomfortable with their baby across their stomachs, try the football hold while still turning your baby's tummy towards you a bit.)

- Relax your wrists. We often try so hard to make sure our baby does not slide away from the breast. But a flexed wrist can push your baby's head down, making it more difficult to swallow. This may also lead to wrist pain that can be easily prevented.[2]

You have probably already heard of positions like the football hold or cross-cradle. There is no right position for holding your baby. You will probably use several at different times. Do what works best for you and your baby, while taking the posture cues above to keep yourself relaxed and in good alignment.

Is My Latch Right?

An improper latch is one of the main issues I see in a new breastfeeding mama. A latch that's not quite right can lead to soreness, pain, and cracked or bleeding nipples. One of the most important things you can do if you are experiencing a lot of discomfort while nursing is to ask for help from a lactation consultant. A proper latch may hurt the first few seconds, but it should not hurt the entire time you nurse.

Is your baby opening their mouth wide like a yawn before latching on to your breast? Do not try to nurse your baby if their mouth is only open a small amount. The latch will not be deep enough and can make you sore. When your baby's mouth is open wide, swoop them into your breast quickly. Bring them to you; do not go to them.

NURSE'S TIP

To get a deeper latch, stroke your baby's top lip with your nipple. This will stimulate them to open their mouth wide like a yawn.

Check your baby for fishy lips. You may need a mirror to see a good angle of their mouths. Both the top and bottom lip should be flared open like a fish. If a lip is tucked under, gently run your finger under it to pop it out. Also look to be sure you can see more of the areola, the dark skin around your nipple, above their mouth than below it. Your baby should be close to your breast with their nose touching or almost touching the breast. Don't worry, if you can see one nostril, your baby is breathing!

You can easily break a latch if it's uncomfortable, or if you are done nursing, by sticking a clean pinky finger in the side of your baby's mouth. Once you are done nursing, your nipples should be round and full looking, not flat or creased. Round and full means your baby was latched properly and deeply enough. Flat or creased means the latch was off and it may lead to nipple trauma.

Is My Baby Getting Enough?

I know it's hard not to wonder if your baby is getting enough milk when you're breastfeeding. I certainly get it, but you typically can trust a full-term, healthy baby's cues. They do a good job of letting you know if they are hungry or satisfied. Once your milk comes in, you should be able to hear your baby swallowing breast milk. Before feeding your breasts will feel full, and after you will notice an obvious softening. Your baby should seem satisfied after feeding. Watch for wet and dirty diapers. You could track these in an app to be sure they are having enough.[3] An evidence-based method would be a weight check. Weighing your baby before feeding and after can give you a definite look into how much milk they are getting.

What Do I Do If My Nipples Are Cracked or Bleeding?

Just because you see cracked or bleeding nipples doesn't mean nursing will not go well for you. It does mean that you need to do some troubleshooting to figure out why this is happening. The most common reason is an ineffective latch. Look at my latch tips to see if there is room for improvement.

QUESTION:
Should I use silver nursing cups?

ANSWER: For the mom with cracked or bleeding nipples, I recommend silver cups for their antibacterial, antifungal properties. These are evidence-backed healing aids, but they are pricey. Not all moms will have these issues nor need silver cups. If you do have nipple trauma, treat it with silver cups, but don't forget to find the source of the problem so it doesn't happen again.

SALT SOAK FOR CRACKED NIPPLES

½ tsp. fine grain Himalayan pink salt   1 cup warm water

1. Wash your hands.
2. Pour the warm water into a mixing bowl and add the salt. Stir until combined. You can also pour the water into two medicine cups.
3. Lean over the bowl or cups, and soak nipples for only three minutes.
4. Rinse with warm water and pat to dry.
5. Apply hand-expressed breast milk, coconut oil, or lanolin.
6. Recommended three times per day for three days.
7. Make a new soak recipe with each use.

Once the nipples are cracked or bleeding, make sure the latch is correct, use the salt soak as written, and use freshly expressed breast milk or silver cups on your nipples. You can continue to breastfeed your baby through this issue, but if it's simply too uncomfortable, only nurse on one side at the next feeding and pump the side that's struggling. Use fresh nursing pads after each session to help prevent any infection.

How Can I Increase My Milk Supply?

Drink Gatorade. No, really. This may be one of the more surprising methods my lactation consultant friends recommend to their patients for increasing milk supply, but it works! Though I could not find studies that touted the benefits of Gatorade on milk supply, breastfeeding professionals swear by it. One reason this may work so well is it helps keep a mother hydrated. Staying hydrated is key to keeping a good milk supply. Most new moms need around 8 cups of water per day, but "drinking to thirst" is the goal. One of the top things to pay attention to is whether you are getting enough fluids during the day. So whether it's Gatorade, Body Armor, or another electrolyte drink, sip it frequently to boost your supply.

Be sure your baby is feeding frequently enough. Breastfeeding is a supply-and-demand system. If your feedings have dropped, so will your supply. Your breasts must be emptied regularly to signal your body to make more milk! Put your baby to the breast often.

There are many ways to increase or maintain your milk supply. Eating certain foods like oatmeal, pumpkin, and garlic have been known to give supply a boost.[4] Lactation cookies and lactation teas are made with ingredients that are shown in studies[5] to increase supply (see my cookie recipe in chapter 10 for a delicious option!). And many supplements are known to give you a boost, like fenugreek, maca root, and marshmallow root. It's always a good idea to check in with your healthcare provider before starting supplements and introduce only one new supplement at a time.

Breast Surgery

If you have a history of breast surgery, it may affect your milk supply. Breast-reduction surgery patients often have trouble with producing enough milk for their babies. It's good to be aware of this so you can create achievable breastfeeding goals. Even a teaspoon of breast milk a day will pass mama's immunities to her baby. Exclusive breastfeeding may not be possible, but large volumes don't have to be the goal.

Breast-enhancement surgery usually has the opposite effects. These mamas tend to have more milk than they need. They often build freezer stashes quickly! Hopefully, if you had breast surgery, your surgeon went over how it may affect breastfeeding. There are several types of surgeries, and each can affect milk ducts differently. If they did not share this information with you, it's not too late to give their office a call and ask questions. Your lactation consultant can also answer questions for you.

Engorgement

I woke up around day four with my first baby with breasts as hard as rocks. I was so sore and thought, *Oh my gosh, is this what breastfeeding is going to feel like?* The answer to my question was no. I was experiencing engorgement. It's normal to get engorged when your mature milk first comes in. This is usually around day three to five for a first-time mama. Your breasts will feel hard and heavy like rocks and will probably be very warm to the touch. But don't worry; this is temporary and usually only lasts around two days. Then your body will adjust. You will have just as much milk as you did, but it will not feel so uncomfortable.

You may find that your baby has a hard time latching on when you are engorged. You can help them out by using warm compresses for a couple of minutes before latching, soaking your breast in warm water for two minutes, or hand expressing a small amount of milk to soften things up for them. This usually does the trick.

To help with your own comfort while engorged, use warm compresses before nursing and cold compresses after nursing. If you are showering, turn your chest away from the water spray. Warm water can stimulate milk production and tell your body to make more, making engorgement worse. You could also take a nonsteroidal anti-inflammatory like ibuprofen if your healthcare provider has approved it. Hang in there, Mama! This should only last a couple of days.

Clogged Milk Duct

I remember waking up the morning of my very first clogged duct. It felt like that side of my boob was so full of milk that it would explode. It caused a feeling of "I've got to get this out!" I nursed my baby, but the clog did not resolve. Sometimes nursing alone will fix it, but not this time.

So I warmed up a compress, massaged the duct, and decided to pump. As I pumped, I used my thumb and gently massaged the duct down towards my nipple (you could also use a lactation massager). Within a few minutes, the clog released, and I was able to empty my breast. Sweet relief!

Sometimes turning your baby to nurse toward the clogged duct can cause it to release. If nursing doesn't seem to be cutting it, use a warm compress and gentle massage (either with your hand or a lactation massager) during nursing. Other times, you may need warm compresses, massage, or a pump to get relief. An NSAID pain reliever (like ibuprofen) is also a good option if your doctor has cleared you for those and you feel it is needed. Sunflower Lecithin is an over-the-counter option for reoccurring clogged ducts that many lactation consultants are now recommending.[6] Though it's uncomfortable, a clogged duct usually unclogs within a couple of nursing or pumping sessions.

QUESTION:
What do I need to know about bottle feeding?

ANSWER: If you want your baby to take a bottle while breastfeeding, begin to offer it around three to five weeks. Starting later than this can lead to bottle refusal. Do paced bottle feedings. Hold the bottle parallel to the floor. This allows baby to be in control of the milk flow. They will draw it out, much like they do out of the breast. Do not forget to pump if your baby takes a bottle instead of the breast.

Pumping

There are so many brands of pumps out there now that it would be impossible for me to cover them all here. But I guarantee you can find a tutorial on YouTube if you need one! Your nurses in the hospital can also help you set up and use your pump, as well as the lactation consultants. If you would like help with it, be sure to ask.

QUESTION:
Are lactation consults covered by insurance?

ANSWER: Under the Affordable Care Act, plans *must* cover breastfeeding support and supplies. This includes lactation consults prenatally and postpartum along with breast pumps. Contact your insurance company about pumps, and look at their online directory for approved providers. If there are none, by law, they must cover your choice of an out-of-network provider.

If you would like to build a milk supply stash because you plan to go back to work, pump one session per day (on top of your normal nursing sessions) for one month before starting your new schedule. The mornings can be a great time for the extra pumping session, as you tend to have the greatest amount of milk in the mornings. Nurse your baby first, then pump what's left. This helps increase your supply and build a freezer stash. Be sure to store your milk, labeled with dates, in a separate bin free from contamination of other foods.

Oh, what a day and age to be a pumping mother! There are so many amazing pumps on the market. From high-end pumps, to wearable to-go pumps, to hand-held manual pumps, there is a pump to fit all lifestyles. You can also find simple, wearable milk-collectors that catch milk leakage, like the Haakaa Ladybugs. If you tend to leak milk, these can help you catch your supply and save it for later. Check with your insurance provider, since many will provide pumps at no or low cost.

HOW LONG TO STORE BREAST MILK

ROOM TEMPERATURE: up to 4 hours

REFRIGERATOR: up to 3 days

THAWED IN FRIDGE: good for 24 hours

THAWED AT ROOM TEMP: good for 2 hours

FREEZER: up to 6 months

Mastitis

Mastitis is a breast infection that usually needs antibiotics to clear up. If you are having pain in one area of the breast, see a red spot, or the red spot feels hot to the touch, you may have mastitis. This usually comes with flu-like symptoms like fever and chills. The number one reason we see mastitis infections is underwire bras. Make sure your nursing bras are underwire free.

If this happens, keep nursing and call your healthcare provider. Cold-turkey quitting nursing will cause a whole host of problems along with all the other discomforts of mastitis. Mastitis will not hurt your baby, and neither will the antibiotics they prescribe you for it.

What If My Milk Supply Has Dropped?

It's common for breastfeeding mothers who have been at it for a couple months to think their milk supply has dropped. It may be true, but it also may not be. Our bodies are excellent adaptors. Even our breasts learn to be efficient, so nursing our babies may not feel like it felt in the early days. We may not leak as much or feel as full.

The best way to find out how your milk supply is doing is to make an appointment with a lactation consultant to have your baby receive a pre- and post-feed weight. Your baby will be weighed before nursing and then again afterward on a highly precise baby scale. This gives you an excellent view of how much your baby is receiving and you can adjust from there.

When I started back to work full time with my first baby, my milk supply tumbled. After seeing Lorraine, my lactation consultant friend, I found my baby was underweight and my milk supply was next to nothing. What do you do when your goal is exclusive breastfeeding but you can't do it? You cry. Then you gather yourself and make new goals. I learned that a teaspoon of breast milk gave my baby all my immune-fighting ability even though it was not much volume. My new goal became pumping enough to give him a small volume each day until we were finished with cold and flu season while transitioning him to a formula that met his immediate nutritional needs.

Of course, it was emotional. It's tempting to feel like a failure when you don't meet your goals, but I was not a failure. I was a good mom willing to change my expectations to meet my baby's needs. I was learning some of my first lessons of motherhood.

NURSE'S TIP

Find a lactation consultant you trust. Many offer prenatal consults, so you can learn and get to know them before you experience any issues. The connection you make will be a lasting resource throughout your breastfeeding journey.

Oversupply

Though undersupply is a common concern, some moms find they have an issue with oversupply. The main reason oversupply happens is overstimulation. Some moms don't realize they are overstimulating. Products that provide gentle suction but are being used for milk collection, like Haakaa's manual pump, send the message to the breast that there is a greater need for milk supply. This, as well as firm massage, can cause an oversupply issue. If you use breast massage for comfort, treat your breast like you are testing an avocado for ripeness. The pressure should be gentle. Using cool compresses following nursing or pumping can also decrease overstimulation and oversupply.

Weaning

Ready to wean? Do it slowly if possible. With my first baby, I had already lost so much of my supply when I weaned that I did not have trouble with pain and clogged ducts. It was not until the third day of weaning that I even felt full for the first time. But if this is not the case for you, begin to drop nursing sessions slowly. Listen to your body. If your breasts feel painful and you need relief, nurse or pump only for a few minutes until you feel better. Do not empty all the way; this signals your body to make more milk. Lactation consultants often advise weaning mothers, "Anything that dries up your sinuses, will dry up your milk too." Wear a supportive, underwire-free bra, like a sports bra, and use cold therapy on your breasts for comfort. And be aware that you will have lots of hormone changes during this process. You may feel emotional or weepy through it.

. . . .

Here's a word of encouragement: If you can make it for the first two weeks of breastfeeding, you can usually make it as long as you want. The first two weeks are a time of great adjustment. This is also the time when most moms experience some kind of issue. If you choose to persist and get help when needed, breastfeeding typically smooths out after two weeks for you and your baby.

You may also have one breast that seems to be your "milk maid." Our right breasts tend to make more milk than our left (though the opposite can be true). You may also notice that your baby tends to favor one side or the other. This is common. Just be sure to rotate the starting sides at each nursing session to give both breasts the opportunity to make the milk they need to.

It's easy to feel some shame if breastfeeding doesn't come naturally like we expect it to. I know I did. I am a postpartum nurse who helps new mothers nurse frequently. I work side by side with lactation consultants, and yet my first two babies had big issues with nursing. I did not want people to know I used a nipple shield or that I had to pump to feed my baby.

Then there are my mamas that bottle feed. Maybe they have a medical reason that they are unable to nurse. Maybe they have personal reasons or circumstances where breastfeeding just isn't going to work for them. The way you feed your baby isn't what makes you a good mom. Choosing what's best for you *is* choosing what's best for your baby too.

The bottom line is that you don't have to share your breastfeeding journey with anyone you are not comfortable with. But you may be surprised to know that most mothers do struggle in some way as a first-time breastfeeding mother. It was not just me, and it is not just you. And it certainly does not make you any less of a mother if breastfeeding has been a process.

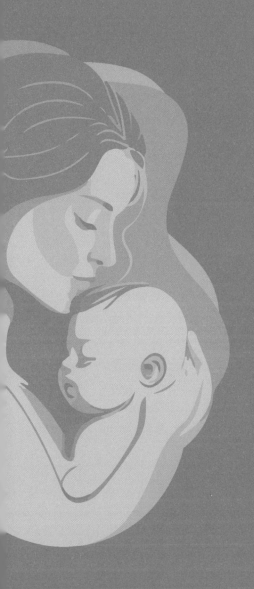

PART TWO

Food

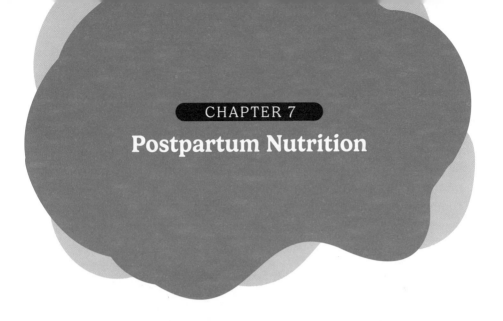

CHAPTER 7

Postpartum Nutrition

O nce again, I was wide awake. I looked at the clock: 4:00 a.m. My baby did not wake me up. He was sound asleep in his little bassinet. It was my stomach—hunger pangs so intense that I thought I would vomit. I had to have food right away. I could not help but feel I was wasting my precious sleep time while satisfying my need for food, but my body was obviously sending me a message. I needed calories.

I learned to keep a protein bar by my bed to minimize my awake time. I would eat as fast as I could so I could hurry back to sleep. My husband would joke with me, "I knew it was 4 a.m. because I could hear the wrapper on that Lärabar!"

Nutrition Guidelines

Throughout pregnancy, women are given clear guidelines for nutrition, but many are left feeling lost in the fourth trimester. In fact, if all you know is that now you can have deli meat and sushi, you are not alone!

There are not many food restrictions in the postpartum world. You can now have the foods that were discouraged in pregnancy. It is still encouraged to eat a healthy diet full of meats, proteins, whole grains, fresh fruits, and veggies. But there are a few changes.

First off, if you are breastfeeding, you need around 500 extra calories every day to meet your and your baby's nutritional needs (hence my 4 a.m. ravenous wakings). These extra calories can be from healthy snacks, extra meal portions, or protein shakes. Realistically, it is going to look like a combination of all these things. If the food you are eating gives you gas, it may give your baby gas, so introduce foods like broccoli and beans slowly.

NURSE'S TIP

Fill your belly with warm meals. Many moms forget to eat meals and end up snacking through the day. Snacks are great, but your body needs more. Aim for one plate or bowl full of a warm meal at least twice per day.

Protein

Exclusively breastfeeding mothers need more protein than other women. Research tells us that exclusively breastfeeding mothers need 1.7 to 1.9 grams of protein per kilogram per day.[1] For my American friends, to find out where this puts you, pull up Google, type in "pounds to kilograms convertor," type in your pounds, and see where you land. Multiply this by 1.7, and this is the minimum amount of protein you need each day. Yikes! I found I usually got half my recommended number. If you are like most women, you don't eat enough protein either. Even mothers who aren't breastfeeding need more protein than other women. Protein helps the postpartum body heal! Adding a healthy protein shake, lean meats, Greek yogurt or beans, lentils, nuts, and chickpeas can help you reach these protein goals. And be sure to eat meals, not just snacks; it's a must.

Galactagogues

Galactagogues are substances or foods known to increase or induce milk supply. These can be beneficial to work into the diet while breastfeeding. Supplements like fenugreek, milk-thistle, and brewer's yeast have long been praised as effective herbal galactagogues. Foods like fennel, oats, alfalfa sprouts, and lentils are also well-known galactagogues. I have a tough time swallowing pills, so I was never consistent with loading up on supplements, but working galactagogue foods into my diet was achievable! Be honest with yourself and do what you know you will do.

GALACTAGOGUES
(FOODS THAT BOOST MILK SUPPLY)

- Oats
- Pumpkin
- Garlic
- Chickpeas
- Ginger
- Papaya
- Dark, leafy greens
- Almonds

Whole Foods

I am a big proponent of eating whole foods as much as possible, postpartum or not. Food is fuel for our bodies. Sara Gottfried, a leading physician in precision medicine and a hormone expert, says, "The food on your fork determines gene expression, hormone levels, immune activity—even stress levels in your gut, your brain, and the rest of your body."[2] Basically, the food we eat matters and determines the health of many of our other functions. If we are mainly eating processed foods, our bodies cannot get the nutrition they need. We begin to feel the effects of it: lack of energy, mood issues, brain fog, and overall blah feelings. If we continue with a poor diet, we know it leads to other big issues like unhealthy weight gain, diabetes, depression, and heart issues.

Making huge dietary changes postpartum can be unrealistic, so work in better choices as you can. That will go a long way. Avoid the processed-food aisles in the grocery store. Replace prepackaged cookies and snacks with homemade items. Look at ingredient lists. Can you pronounce them? Choose products that are non-GMO and organic when you can. Swap processed cereals for oatmeal. Go for grass-fed or grass-finished, organic meats when you can. Backyard eggs are another highly nutritious food option.

I understand it's not feasible for everyone to spend large amounts of money on super healthy foods, and I also never wish to place the burden on your shoulders of needing to do this when you are not able. I certainly remember seasons of my life when grass-finished meats were not in the budget. Work in the best choices you can. Items like organic tomato sauce and organic peanut butter are now available at reasonable prices. Check out the dirty dozen list each year and choose a couple of items you could replace with organic.[3] This helps you get better food on your fork without breaking your budget.

Collagen and Omegas

Collagen is wonderful to add to the postpartum diet. It gives a boost of protein but also helps your tissues mend and heal. It is great for your nails and hair too! Omega-3 fatty acids may be in the vitamins you are taking, but you can also add wild salmon to your diet to get a great boost of these. There is also evidence that Omega-3 fatty acids help with postpartum depression.[4]

Many of us simply do not get the minerals our body needs from the foods we eat. Our nation's farming techniques have stripped many minerals from the soil our veggies grow in. Switching out part of your table salt to Himalayan pink salt gives you some extra minerals too. Taking an Epsom salt bath also gives you needed magnesium, and bonus: It can help you relax and sleep better! (Most healthcare providers recommend waiting to take a bath until four weeks postpartum.)

Alcohol

For centuries, folklore has told us that drinking alcohol regularly while breastfeeding increases breast milk. Science tells us otherwise. Though occasionally drinking alcohol is safe for a nursing mother and will not affect her baby or her milk supply, drinking it daily actually decreases a mom's milk supply.[5] Overall, drinking alcohol in moderation is considered safe for the postpartum mother (unlike in pregnancy). Current research tells us that alcohol levels peak in the breast milk between 30-60 minutes after consuming the drink, and it's best to wait two hours before nursing again after drinking. So, if you want a drink, nurse first, drink second. Professionals no longer recommend pumping and dumping after a drink.[6]

The main issue with having an occasional drink is it leads to dehydration. A breastfeeding mother does not need to be dehydrated! If you choose to have a drink, be sure to add extra water intake so your body has enough to make milk. New mothers should never drink alcohol to the point that they are impaired. And it is best to drink alcohol occasionally, not daily. I recommend the maximum amount consumed should be one to two drinks per week, and I never recommend a nursing mother drink more than one drink at her dinner or outing. In fact, anything that impairs your ability to care for your baby needs to be avoided. This could put your baby's safety at risk, and nothing is worth that.

········WAYS TO SNEAK IN NUTRITION········

- Keep a full water bottle by your normal nursing spot.
- Make a smoothie each day. Add protein powder and Greek yogurt.

- Add a scoop of collagen powder to your morning coffee.

- Pack several easy-to-grab fridge bento boxes with cheese, nuts, and pretzels.

- Make a basket of high-protein snacks like bars, beef sticks, and nuts.

- Or ask someone else to help you with these.

Caffeine

It is also believed that caffeine drinks are safe while nursing.[7] Most experts recommend no more than two cups of caffeine per day. I personally recommend you have these earlier in the day so it does not put your baby at risk of wanting to stay up and party halfway through the night. Again, be sure to drink extra water if drinking things that dehydrate your body, like coffee.

Hydration

Proper water intake is important to not only the breastfeeding mother but also the postpartum mother. Hydration helps your bodily systems function better, which leads to better recovery and healing. It can also help rid you of extra fluids from pregnancy and helps control swelling. As a breastfeeding mother who gave birth in the summertime, I drank 12 cups of water every day and sometimes more. If you are thirsty, drink water.

Tired of water all the time? It is safe to work in electrolyte drinks as well. Things like Bodyarmor SuperDrink and Gatorade can give you a hydration boost if you need something other than water. Making your own Mama-Ade can be a great natural, homemade alternative as well.

MAMA-ADE RECIPE

2 cups pressed coconut water ⅓ cup fresh lime juice 2 T. honey dissolved in 2 T. hot water

¼ tsp. Celtic sea salt

1 cup filtered water

METHOD

1. In a 32-ounce mason jar, mix coconut water, water, lime juice, sea salt, and honey syrup.

2. Refrigerate until ready to drink.

3. Doubles or triples well. Stir before drinking. Hydrates, replenishes electrolytes, and helps reduce adrenaline.

Recipe courtesy of Jeanna McNeil, ByDesign Birth Doula

Vitamins and Supplements

I encourage you to continue taking prenatal vitamins for as long as you are breastfeeding. If you are not breastfeeding, take your prenatal vitamins for six weeks. You can swap out prenatal vitamins for postnatal vitamins. A postnatal multivitamin from a good source (think non-GMO and whole food) would be very helpful for you to continue throughout your fourth trimester.[8] Other supplements you may consider are milk-boosting herbs like fenugreek, biotin (to help with hair loss), and zinc (to help with wound healing and immunity support) if they are not already included in your vitamins. If your healthcare provider recommends an iron supplement, look for one made from whole foods.[9] This will help your body absorb it better and also prevent unwanted constipation.

SIGNS OF IRON DEFICIENCY

- Dizziness
- Vertigo
- Pale skin
- Low energy

- Breathlessness
- Racing heart/ palpitations

If you experience these signs, work in high-iron foods and call your healthcare provider.

• • • • • • • • • • •

A little bit of effort toward healthy eating can go a long way. If these recommendations are new to you, don't worry about doing all of them at one time. Pick one or two to start with and work them into your new routine. Before you know it, they will feel like normal life, and you can work in a couple more. Each healthy choice you make can gain momentum that leads to other healthy choices. Your body will thank you for every one!

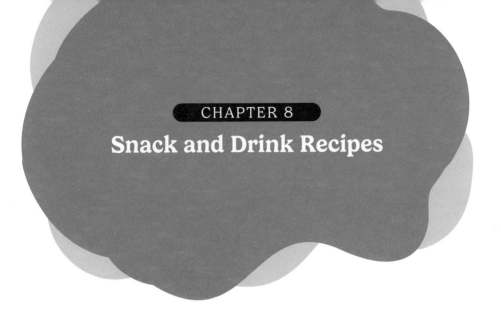

CHAPTER 8

Snack and Drink Recipes

These are some of my favorite recipes for a new mom. They can satisfy a sweet tooth while also giving your body a good boost of needed nutrients. I added nutritional facts for you, but keep in mind, you do not need to be calorie counting as a postpartum mom. Focus more on choosing whole foods, warm meals, and protein-rich snacks.

Food is a love language in itself in the fourth trimester. Have some people offered to help you? Take them up on it and ask them to make you some of these recipes.

COPYCAT PERFECT BARS

. . . .

Easy to make, delicious, and one of my go-to protein snacks!

Prep Time: 10 minutes   *Fridge Time:* 30 minutes to 2 hours

1½ cups creamy organic peanut butter*

½ cup honey

1½ cup nonfat dry milk powder†

½ cup semisweet chocolate chips

METHOD

1. In a large bowl, combine the peanut butter and honey together. Stir well. Add the dry milk powder and mix until completely smooth. This can also be mixed in a food processor if you don't want to stir by hand.

2. With clean fingers, press mixture into a 9 x 13-inch pan.

3. Lightly press chocolate chips into the top of the bars. Feel free to fold a few tablespoons of chocolate chips into the batter if you would like.

4. Cut the bars into 16 rectangles and place them into the refrigerator.

5. These bars can be eaten immediately but will have a softer texture. For a firm "Perfect Bar" texture refrigerate for at least 30 minutes before eating.

Servings: 16

Nutrition Facts (1 of 16 bars): Calories: 225, Total Fat: 13g, Saturated Fat: 3g, Total Carbs: 22, Dietary Fiber: 3g, Sugar: 17g, Protein: 8g

---

* An organic almond butter or sunflower butter can be substituted for the peanut butter.

† Can't have dairy? Try one of these alternatives: cashew milk powder, soy milk powder, or coconut milk powder. All these can be substituted for milk powder at a 1:1 ratio.

NO-BAKE OAT PROTEIN BITES

I could eat this by the spoonful! If you like the taste of boiled or no-bake cookies, you will love these. These bites offer a great protein boost. Feel free to substitute other nut butters for the peanut butter if you wish.

Prep Time: 20 minutes   *Freeze Time:* 15 minutes

2½ cups organic rolled oats*

⅓ cup honey

1 scoop of your favorite protein powder† (I use Garden of Life Organic Protein in chocolate)

⅔ cup plus 1 T. organic peanut butter

⅓ cup extra virgin coconut oil

METHOD

1. Place oats and protein powder in a bowl. Stir together.
2. Heat a small saucepan over low heat. Mix the peanut butter, coconut oil, and honey in the saucepan and heat until smooth. Do not boil.
3. Pour peanut butter sauce over the bowl of oats. Mix well.
4. Press onto a wax-paper-lined 9 x 13-inch pan or roll into walnut-sized balls. Freeze for 15 minutes. If you didn't shape the bites into balls, cut them into 32 squares. Refrigerate your oat bites until you are ready to eat them.

Variation: Throw a handful of semisweet chocolate chips into your peanut butter sauce. Stir until melted. These taste just like my mom's boiled cookies recipe but without the flour and refined sugar.

Servings: 32

Nutrition Facts (1 of 32 No-Bake Oat Protein Bites): Calories: 97, Total Fat: 6g, Saturated Fat: 2g, Total Carbs: 9g, Dietary Fiber: 1g, Sugar: 3g, Protein: 3g

---

* Quick oats can also be substituted but will give the bites a smoother texture.

† The protein powder can be omitted if desired.

MOTHER'S CHAI TEA LATTE

I have a confession to make. I do not like licorice. I am a big fan of the ingredients of Traditional Medicinals' brand of Mother's Milk Tea but not the taste. So I set out to create a recipe I enjoyed and would still give me the benefits of the herbs in the tea. I hope you enjoy it too!

Prep Time: 15 minutes

1 Traditional Medicinals Mother's Milk Lactation Tea Bag	¼ cup Tazo Classic Chai Concentrate*	1 tsp. honey
¼ cup water	1 cup oat milk	Sprinkle of cinnamon and turmeric

METHOD

1. Heat water to boiling. I use the stove top, but a microwave or electric kettle works too. Place the tea bag in an 11-ounce coffee mug and pour water over the top. Cover and allow to steep for ten minutes.

2. Meanwhile, heat the Tazo concentrate and oat milk until steaming hot, but not boiling. Slowly pour it into the mug. Remove the tea bag.

3. Stir in honey, cinnamon, and turmeric. Sip and enjoy your moment!

Servings: 1

Nutrition Facts for Mother's Chai Tea Latte: Calories: 170, Total Fat: 5g, Saturated Fat: 0.5g, Total Carbs: 28.3g, Dietary Fiber: 1.5g, Sugar: 20.7g, Protein: 2.1g

---

* Contains approximately 20mg of caffeine which is equal to the amount of caffeine in less than ¼ cup of coffee.

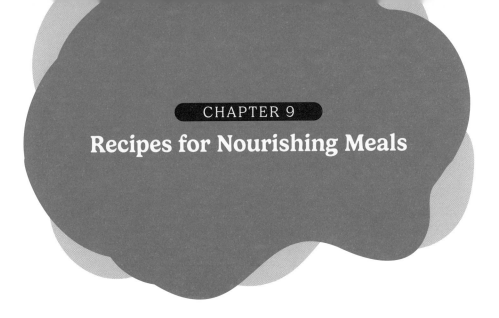

CHAPTER 9

Recipes for Nourishing Meals

I have a small amount of catering experience in my past. Nothing huge. Mostly small events and parties for people who love my cooking. At one time, a booth within another shop gave me the chance to sell my cinnamon rolls and hot chocolate bombs. All these things gave me opportunities to work on something I love to do: cook.

I attribute this love to my great-grandmother. She was a true Southern cook. Though she had a low income, she cooked well with what she had. My favorite were her biscuits. To this day, I have never had one that came close to hers.

She would always begin cooking dinner at 3:00 p.m. Can you believe that? Very few of us could manage that today with our busy schedules. If you have the time, that's great, but I'm a firm believer in all types of recipes: the kind that take hours and the kind that take minutes. Both are appropriate on certain days.

The following are some of my favorite recipes tailored for the nutrition needs of the postpartum mama. Some are quick, and some take all day. The recipes that take all day are great to make *for* a new mama. You will notice I often opt for organic ingredients, especially when they are affordable. If organic is not within the budget, substitute with nonorganic ingredients. The recipe will still be delicious!

I believe food can be healing—not only to our recovering bodies but also to our souls. That's why when I feel sad, my mom can make her cheesy eggs and it lifts my spirit. I hope you find these recipes to be yummy, soothing, and just what you need on your journey of recovery.

SLOW-COOKER BONE BROTH ROAST WITH VEGGIES

This is one of my favorite recipes to make for a new mama. It's packed with nourishing ingredients and is comforting to eat! I am using store-bought bone broth to save some time, but I include how to make your own beef bone broth at the bottom of the recipe.

Prep Time: 15 minutes   *Cook Time:* 10 hours

1 (2 lb.) grass-fed, chuck roast

Salt and pepper to taste

4 organic russet potatoes, rinsed and unpeeled, cut into bite-size pieces

6 organic carrots, rinsed and unpeeled, cut into pieces

1 cup beef bone broth*

2 tsp. Better Than Bouillon Roasted Beef Base

2 cloves garlic, smashed

Optional gravy (recipe below)

METHOD

1. Place the chuck roast in your slow cooker. Lightly salt and pepper it. Put in the potatoes, carrots, and garlic.

2. Mix the Better than Bouillon Base in the cup of beef broth. Pour evenly over the veggies.

3. Cover and cook on low for 10 hours until the roast is tender and shreds easily with a fork.

OPTIONAL GRAVY

2 T. butter	½ cup whole milk	1 T. Better Than Bouillon
2 T. all-purpose flour	½ cup water	Roasted Beef Base

METHOD

1. When the roast is finished cooking, heat butter in a skillet over medium heat. Once melted, whisk in the flour. Whisk until it is bubbly and golden, about two minutes.

2. Meanwhile, in a separate cup, stir Better Than Bouillon into the milk and water. Slowly stir this liquid into the butter and flour roux. Whisk constantly until bubbling and thick. Ladle over the roast and serve immediately.

*TO MAKE YOUR OWN BEEF BROTH

1. Use three pounds of beef bones, like oxtail, knuckle, or shank. Preheat your oven to 450° F and roast the bones on a large baking sheet for 40 minutes, flipping over halfway through.

2. Place the bones into a large stockpot, and add one onion, without the skin, cut into fourths. Then add two celery stalks cut in half, two carrots cut in half, four garlic cloves, and two teaspoons of salt. Cover with 12 cups of water.

3. Bring to a boil and reduce heat to a low simmer. Cover and simmer for 12 hours, occasionally skimming off the foam or gunk that surfaces. If the vegetables or beef become uncovered with water, add more.

4. Cool down and strain with a fine mesh strainer or cheese cloth. Do not forget to put a large pot or bowl under the strainer! Discard the bones and vegetables. Store broth in the refrigerator for one week or freeze for up to three months.

Servings of Roast: 6

Nutrition Facts for Slow-Cooker Bone Broth Roast with Optional Gravy per serving: Calories: 546, Total Fat: 31g, Saturated Fat: 13g, Total Carbs: 29g, Dietary Fiber: 3g, Sugar: 6g, Protein: 38g

CREAMY TOMATO BASIL SOUP

Oh, so good! This tomato basil soup is simple to make and ready in 30 minutes. Add a fresh loaf of sourdough bread, and it makes for a comforting meal. It's a family favorite.

Prep Time: 10 minutes   *Cook Time:* 30 minutes

1 (28 oz.) can organic crushed tomatoes with basil	1 (14 oz.) can organic tomato sauce	10 basil leaves
	1 cup organic chicken broth	1 cup organic heavy cream
	2 tsp. brown sugar	½ cup shredded parmesan

METHOD

1. In a medium saucepan, add the crushed tomatoes, tomato sauce, brown sugar (cuts the acidity) and chicken broth. Bring to a boil and reduce to low heat. Simmer for 25 minutes.

2. In the meantime, cut the basil into strips.

3. After the soup has simmered for 25 minutes, turn off the heat. Add the basil. If you wish to puree the soup, you can do it at this point. Add cream. Stir until incorporated.

4. Ladle into bowls, top with parmesan, and serve immediately.

5. Can be refrigerated for three days.

Servings: 6

Nutrition Facts for Creamy Tomato Basil Soup per serving: Calories: 227, Total Fat: 15g, Saturated Fat: 10g, Total Carbs: 18g, Dietary Fiber: 3g, Sugar: 9g, Protein: 9g

MAKE-IT-FOR-A-NEW-MAMA LASAGNA

This takes a little time, but it is so good! I have not found a lasagna yet that competes with it. Because of the preparation and cooking time, it is great to have someone make this for you, or to make it and freeze it before your due date. Once you have had this, you will never want to go back to frozen lasagna!

Prep Time: 30 minutes　　　　*Cook Time:* 2 hours, 30 minutes

1 lb. mild Italian sausage	1 (28 oz.) can organic crushed tomatoes with basil	1 tsp. salt
½ lb. lean ground beef		1 tsp. Italian seasoning
1 small yellow onion, chopped		12 lasagna noodles
2 cloves garlic, chopped	2 (14 oz.) cans organic tomato sauce	16 oz. ricotta cheese
1 T. white sugar	2 T. chopped parsley	1 egg
	½ tsp. dried basil	18 slices mozzarella cheese
		½ cup shredded parmesan

METHOD

1. Crumble and cook sausage, beef, onion, and garlic in a Dutch oven or large saucepan over medium heat until well browned.

2. Stir in sugar, crushed tomatoes, tomato sauce, basil, and Italian seasoning. (If you wish, add ½ teaspoon fennel here. I have found many who do not care for fennel, so I opt to leave it out.) Cover and simmer for 1½ hours. Stir occasionally.

3. Bring a large pot of water to a boil. Add lasagna noodles and cook for nine minutes, while stirring occasionally. Drain noodles and rinse with cold water to stop the cooking process.

4. In a medium mixing bowl, mix ricotta cheese, egg, 1 teaspoon salt, and the parsley. Set aside.

5. Preheat the oven to 375° F.

6. To assemble lasagna: Spread 1½ cups of meat sauce on the bottom of a 9 x 13-inch dish. Place six noodles on top. Spread the noodles with half of the ricotta mixture. Top with six mozzarella cheese

slices. Pour another 1½ cups of meat sauce on top and sprinkle with a handful of parmesan.

7. Repeat these layers. Let the last layer be the last of your shredded parmesan and six mozzarella slices. Cover the lasagna with foil. Leave some room between the foil and lasagna so the cheese does not stick, or spray the foil with nonstick spray.

8. Bake in the preheated oven 35 minutes. Remove the foil and bake an additional 15 minutes. Allow the lasagna to rest 15 minutes before serving. It will hold together better.

HOW TO FREEZE LASAGNA

If you are making this recipe to be frozen, prepare and bake it in an aluminum foil pan. Allow the lasagna to cool completely and cover the entire dish in plastic wrap. Wrap the top in aluminum foil. Can be frozen for up to three months.

HOW TO REHEAT FROZEN LASAGNA

Thaw the lasagna in the fridge overnight. Remove plastic wrap and replace the aluminum foil cover on top. Preheat oven to 350° F and bake the lasagna for 45 minutes. Test the middle of the lasagna to be sure it is bubbling hot. If not, put it back in the oven for another 10 minutes. Continue this until it is piping hot.

Servings: 10

Nutrition Facts for Make-It-For-A-New-Mama Lasagna per serving: Calories: 550, Total Fat: 35g, Saturated Fat: 12g, Total Carbs: 48g, Dietary Fiber: 6g, Sugar: 13g, Protein: 32g

TURKEY CRUNCH WRAP WITH MIXED GREENS

I love a good turkey wrap! This one is packed with flavor and nutritious ingredients that can help a new mom meet her daily needs. It is also easy to throw together quickly. It's a lunch you can feel good about!

Prep Time: 5 minutes   *Cook Time:* 2 minutes

- 1 flatbread (I use Joseph's Lavash Bread)
- 1 wedge The Laughing Cow Creamy Spicy Pepper Jack Cheese
- 2 tsp. Chick-fil-A Sauce
- 2 tsp. chopped red onions, optional
- Sliced tomato, optional
- 6 slices of your favorite deli turkey
- 1 cup organic mixed greens
- 2 tsp. extra virgin olive oil

METHOD

1. Heat a large skillet over medium heat.

2. While the skillet heats, lay the flatbread out horizontally. Spread the wedge of Laughing Cow over the flatbread, being sure to add some to the left short edge so when you roll it up, it stays together. Add the Chick-fil-A sauce and spread around. Sprinkle on the red onions if desired.

3. Add your sliced turkey to the middle area of the wrap. Top with tomato slices.

4. At the right end of the flatbread, opposite the end with the Laughing Cow cheese edge, add the cup of mixed greens. Keeping the greens at the end and starting your roll there, keeps them fresh and not wilted.

5. Starting at the side of the flatbread with your greens, roll your wrap up, pressing gently at the end to help the Laughing Cow spread keep the roll together.

6. Add the olive oil to your hot skillet. Place your wrap in the skillet for one minute. Adjust the temperature if you need to. Flip the wrap and cook for one minute more. Serve immediately.

7. Feel free to get creative with the fillings—bacon, basil, cranberry sauce, avocado, or peaches are all options that can keep your wrap from getting boring and could be a great way to pack in some extra nutrition.

Servings: 1

Nutrition Facts for Turkey Crunch Wrap with Mixed Greens per serving (includes tomatoes and onions): Calories: 545, Total Fat: 29g, Saturated Fat: 4g, Total Carbs: 26g, Dietary Fiber: 4g, Sugar: 7g, Protein: 36g

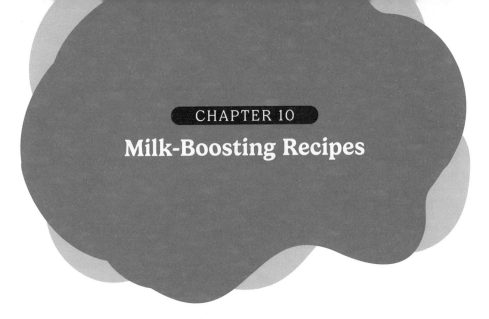

CHAPTER 10

Milk-Boosting Recipes

I was sitting in a mothers' breastfeeding room about to teach a class the first time I found out about lactation cookies. *What a great idea*, I thought. I have known about galactagogues—foods, herbs, and supplements that boost milk supply—for a long time. I tried one and muttered, "This is super convenient, but I bet I can make a homemade version that hits the cookie craving better."

I am really thankful for these companies that have brought products to the market for breastfeeding mothers. There was a time when there were none. For those who don't cook or who don't have support people to cook for them, these are great options.

You already know I enjoy cooking. So when I find something I feel is a good idea or that blows my taste buds away, I challenge myself to see if I can create a version at home.

All these milk-boosting recipes are created from those challenges. They had to pass my own taste tests, as well as my husband and children's. (Kids will not lie about the taste of food.) I am happy with the results, and I hope you will be too! Non-breastfeeding people can partake in these recipes, though you won't want them to. They don't contain hormones and won't cause milk production in anyone not already nursing.

Happy breastfeeding, and happy snacking!

LACTATION OATMEAL CHOCOLATE CHIP COOKIES

You would never know these were lactation cookies if I didn't tell you. Soft, delicious oatmeal cookies packed with chocolate chips that also give your milk supply a boost? Yes, please!

Prep Time: 15 minutes   *Cook Time:* 8 minutes

7 T. butter, at room
  temperature
⅓ cup light brown sugar
¼ cup white sugar
1 egg

½ tsp. vanilla extract
½ cup all-purpose flour
5 T. brewer's yeast
3 T. ground flaxseed

½ tsp. baking soda
¼ tsp. salt
1½ cups organic rolled oats
1 cup semisweet chocolate
  chips

METHOD

1. Preheat oven to 350° F.

2. In a large mixing bowl, cream together butter and sugars until fluffy.

3. Beat in the egg and vanilla.

4. Add the flour, brewer's yeast, flaxseed, baking soda, and salt. Combine well.

5. Fold in the oats. Fold in the chocolate chips.

6. Drop by tablespoonful onto an ungreased cookie sheet. Bake for eight to nine minutes until the cookies are golden and the center is set. Allow them to cool a few minutes before moving them to your storage container.

7. Store in a sealed container at room temperature for five days.

Makes approximately 24 cookies

Nutrition Facts (2 Lactation Oatmeal Chocolate Chip Cookies): Calories: 296, Total Fat: 14g, Saturated Fat: 8g, Total Carbs: 40g, Dietary Fiber: 4g, Sugar: 22g, Protein: 6g

PUMPKIN SPICE LACTATION COOKIES

These are simply delightful! Packed with favorite fall flavors plus milk-boosting ingredients, these will satisfy your cookie cravings.

Prep Time: 15 minutes   *Cook Time:* 12 minutes

½ cup butter, softened
1 cup organic pumpkin
  puree
1 cup white sugar
½ cup brown sugar
1 large egg
2 cups all-purpose flour

5 T. brewer's yeast
3 T. ground flaxseed
1 tsp. baking soda
1 tsp. baking powder
¼ tsp. salt
2 tsp. ground cinnamon

½ tsp. nutmeg
½ tsp. cloves

OPTIONAL ICING
1 cup powdered sugar
2 T. milk

A LOADED OPTION

Stir in 1 cup rolled oats, ½ cup coconut flakes, and ½ cup chopped pecans after step 3 and before dropping by tablespoonfuls onto a baking sheet. Proceed with the directions as written.

METHOD

1. Preheat oven to 350° F.

2. Cream butter and pumpkin together in a large mixing bowl.

3. Add the sugars and mix well. Stir in the egg.

4. Add the flour, brewer's yeast, flaxseed, baking soda, baking powder, salt, cinnamon, nutmeg, and cloves to the butter mixture. Stir all together.

5. Drop by tablespoonfuls onto an ungreased baking sheet. Bake for 12 minutes or until the centers are set. While the cookies are baking and cooling, make the icing if desired. Allow to cool before drizzling icing over the cookies and storing in an airtight container at room temperature for 3 days.

Makes approximately 36 cookies
Nutrition Facts (2 Pumkin Spice Lactation Cookies with icing): Calories: 222, Total Fat: 6g, Saturated Fat: 3g, Total Carbs: 39g, Dietary Fiber: 2g, Sugar: 25g, Protein: 4g

MILK-BOOSTING PROTEIN BARS

Similar to the Perfect Bar, this protein bar tastes great but also boasts the added benefit of milk-boosting abilities. This makes it the perfect choice for the breastfeeding mother.

Prep Time: 10 minutes

1½ cups organic, creamy peanut butter*

½ cup honey

1 cup instant, dry milk powder†

2 scoops of lactation protein powder, like Boobie Body

½ cup semisweet chocolate chips

METHOD

1. In a large bowl, combine the peanut butter and honey together. Stir well. Add the dry milk powder and lactation protein powder. Mix until completely smooth.

2. With clean hands, press mixture into a 9 x 13-inch pan.

3. Lightly press chocolate chips into the top of the bars. Feel free to fold a few tablespoons of chocolate chips into the batter if you would like. Cut the bars into 16 rectangles and place them into the refrigerator.

These bars can be eaten immediately but will have a softer texture. For a familiar firm, Perfect Bar texture, refrigerate for at least 30 minutes before eating. This protein bar recipe can also be mixed in a food processor if you don't want to stir by hand.

Servings: 16 bars

Nutrition Facts for Milk-Boosting Protein Bars (1 of 16 bars): Calories: 232, Total Fat: 14g, Saturated Fat: 3g, Total Carbs: 22g, Dietary Fiber: 4g, Sugar: 16g, Protein: 10g

---

* An organic almond butter or sunflower butter can be substituted for the peanut butter.

† An alternative substitution is cashew milk powder, soy milk powder, or coconut milk powder in a 1:1 ratio.

NO-DAIRY PUMPKIN MUFFINS

Prep Time: 15 minutes   *Bake Time:* 18 minutes

1 (14 oz.) can of organic pumpkin puree

½ cup organic virgin or extra virgin coconut oil

⅓ cup white sugar

⅓ cup brown sugar

2 large eggs

¼ cup almond milk

1 cup all-purpose flour

½ cup almond flour

3 T. ground flaxseed

1 tsp. baking soda

1½ tsp. ground cinnamon

1 tsp. pumpkin pie spice

¼ tsp. ground ginger

¼ tsp. salt

1 cup organic rolled oats

½ cup organic unsweetened coconut flakes

½ cup semisweet chocolate chips

METHOD

1. Preheat oven to 375° F.

2. Mix the pumpkin puree and coconut oil together in a large mixing bowl. (If the coconut oil needs to be softened, heat in a saucepan over low heat until just melted.) Stir in the white and brown sugar. Add the eggs and almond milk and mix until incorporated.

3. In a separate bowl, mix the all-purpose flour, almond flour, flaxseed, baking soda, cinnamon, pumpkin pie spice, ginger, and salt.

4. Pour the dry ingredients into the wet ingredients and mix until just combined. Do not over mix or you will get tough muffins.

5. Add the oats, coconut flakes, and chocolate chips. Gently fold into batter until just combined.

6. Lightly grease a muffin tin. Spoon batter into the muffin cups until three quarters full. Bake for 18 minutes. Allow to cool for 10 minutes before removing the muffins from the pan.

7. Store in an airtight container for three days or refrigerate for one week.

Servings: 24 muffins

Nutrition Facts for No-Dairy Pumpkin Muffins per serving (1 of 24 muffins): Calories: 154, Total Fat: 9g, Saturated Fat: 6g, Total Carbs: 17g, Dietary Fiber: 2g, Sugar: 9g, Protein: 2g

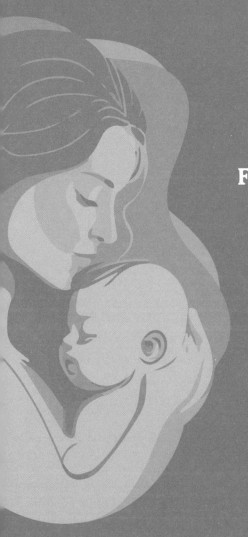

PART THREE

Feelings and Fears

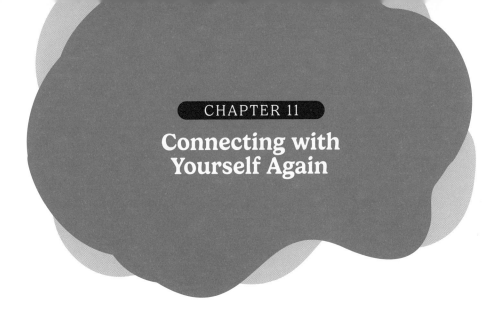

Connecting with Yourself Again

I will never forget sitting down for dinner one evening with my family. The kids were bickering with each other, and my husband casually mentioned a spice he would like to have to make the meal more to his taste. For some reason, that did it.

I slammed my hands down on the table as a scream erupted out of me. It closely resembled a roar. A roar-scream, maybe? I walked into the kitchen and out the back door. My husband sat there, stunned.

I paced back and forth. I had surprised myself. "What just happened?" I muttered.

My default has always been to be what I like to call an emotional stuffer. Take the little bother, the irritation, the hurt, the feelings, and stuff them down with the belief that it dissolves and melts away somewhere inside. Maybe you can relate.

But then something unexpected happens. What we thought we had dealt with erupts like Mount Krakatoa at what appears to be the smallest comment. The eruption then causes a tsunami reaction of shame and disgust with ourselves. *How could I do that? How could I say that? I'm a terrible mom. How can I not be thankful for my family?*

But we are not bad people. What appears to be anger could actually be overwhelm, resentment, overstimulation, exhaustion, grief, or hurt. Or, more than likely, it is a combination of several of these things.

It is a beautiful thing if the person we share our lives with can see beneath the surface of our anger and help us pinpoint the real need. But not every spouse has learned this tool quite yet. Let's be honest: Many of us are still learning this too. And many moms are going at this thing alone, without a solid support system.

Ultimately, though, it is our job to peek into the depths of our own souls and determine what the problem is and identify the need we have. No one can magically read our minds. It is more likely we will be met with understanding if we can form words around what's happening inside of us.

For me, that memorable night reflected something that had been off-kilter for a while. It showed a woman who had begun to believe she was nothing more than the roles she was filling. A full-time mom, a full-time nurse, a wife, a schedule planner, a cook, and a maid. Who I really was, outside of my daily roles and tasks, felt unseen.

I had lost myself. And it felt like others had lost sight of me too.

It's so easy to find ourselves in this place in motherhood. It most often begins postpartum. What starts as vigilance over meeting our baby's needs and often neglecting our own (which is a natural occurrence in the beginning), turns into always meeting our family's needs and leaving ours out to dry. I often read that when our babies begin to discover their own hands, they are beginning to realize they are different than us. It marks the end of the fourth trimester. It's so important that as our baby begins to emerge into their own identities, we do as well.

Connecting to ourselves again is a big deal. We have probably all known women who were married, had kids, raised the kids, and then seemed to lose their minds once the kids were grown. But we know good and well, women do not just lose their minds. More often than not, it is a slow descent from losing sight of who we are or who our spouse is. This can happen when all we are is solely wrapped up in meeting the needs of our children. It is not good for us or for them.

Connecting With Yourself

The term *self-care* has been so overused that many folks roll their eyes when they hear it. But caring for yourself is a big deal. It sends the message to your own heart that, "Yes, my family is valuable, but I am too."

Don't just rush over that part. You are valuable. Not only because you carried, birthed, and sustained life, but because of who you are. You are valuable without children, with children, married, single, or divorced.

I pray that you have people in your life who are surrounding you and meeting your needs in such a vulnerable time, but also that you would know that ultimately there is a God who loves you, created you, and will meet every need you have. I really do believe that.

Self-Regulation

One start to connecting with our own bodies again is through self-regulation practice. We are not powerful enough to change the entire world around us, but we are powerful enough to regulate our nervous system and how we respond to what happens. Many people are dominated by their sympathetic nervous system, or at least easily controlled by it. This is the fight, flight, freeze, or fawn system. Sympathetic nervous system dominance is easy to live with if we are not aware of it and if we do not work to step into our parasympathetic nervous system (our calm system).

Turn your attention to your body for a minute. Do you feel comfortable? Do you notice any tight muscles? Can you purposefully relax them? Most of us are holding tightness in parts of our bodies without ever even realizing it. And we have trained ourselves to do this, many of us from childhood. When we become body aware, we will notice how our muscles respond in certain situations.

For example, if your husband's voice tone begins to climb, or your baby will not stop crying, or you just spilled the milk all over the floor, your body usually has a response. And it's probably for a reason you don't remember. More than likely you have had that response for years.

Once we're aware of what our bodies are doing, we can give them what they need. Let me sidestep for just a moment here and add a gentle reminder: Your body is your friend. It's easy for us to fight against our bodies in different ways and come to the belief that we are somehow on a different side than our bodies are. I know I experienced this when I felt frustrated that my body was not losing weight with my third baby the way it had with my first. The same happened when my breast milk dried up when my goal was to exclusively breastfeed. I had a mentality of "me versus my body," and it was all wrong.

Our bodies are designed to adjust, accommodate, and do what we ask of them. If our bodies don't seem to be fitting our expectations, it may be time to evaluate our expectations and determine if they are what we truly need. My body has gifted me the ability to carry and birth three children. It has allowed me to work as a nurse, try different workout methods, heal when I get sick, rock my children, and play with them as they grew. Forming a friendship with our bodies can bring such peace.

Softening

I told you earlier to turn your attention to your body and notice any tight muscles. Let's try it again. Do you have any? (I do.) Focus on those for a moment. Begin to breathe deeply and slowly and count to five. As you do, soften the tight muscles. One. Two. Three. Four. Five. Continue moving on with your day and check in again in 15 minutes. Are the muscles tight again? Probably so. Go ahead and soften again for five seconds.

Dr. J. Eric Gentry, a leader in the study and treatment of traumatic stress and compassion fatigue, teaches this technique to clients and professionals alike. As he so wisely reminds people, this takes practice. You may do it 200 times a day and find your muscles are tight each time. It simply goes to show you're experiencing sympathetic nervous system dominance, but we have the power to change that in ourselves. He states, "You cannot experience anxiety in a body that is in the parasympathetic nervous system."[1] Though it takes intentional work, purposefully softening our bodies can help us connect back to our calm nervous system again.

Sensory Touch

Often in motherhood, we can feel like our bodies are not our own. Postpartum, we are nursing babies, leaking milk, bleeding, swollen, hurting, and morphing back to our prepregnant size. It's also common to feel we are attending to needs other than ours all day and night. We slip into motions, almost performing out of what we know to do instead of who we are.

Taking a few moments several times a week to connect once again to our own bodies can help. The following exercise sounds elementary, but sometimes it's just what we need to refocus. Sitting in a quiet room with eyes closed, take three deep, slow breaths. With your right hand, touch your left arm and say out loud, "This is my arm." Touch your shoulder and say, "This is my shoulder." Move to your neck, then your other shoulder and your other arm. Touch your feet and say, "These are my feet."

It may be helpful to say your name as you do this. When I feel very disconnected from myself, I will say, "Rachel, this is your hand." It seems to better join my body back to my heart.

Your body and emotions are trying to speak to you. They are part of your team. Don't be quick to shoo them away. Turn softly in toward yourself and listen to what you need. Taking a few minutes each day to attend to your own needs helps connect you back to yourself during this transition in the fourth trimester.

CHAPTER 12

Postpartum Blues Versus Postpartum Depression

As I paced back and forth through my living room clutching my two-week-old baby to my chest, tears streamed down my face and dripped off my cheek. My husband was wide-eyed at my emotions. I was not usually an overly emotional person. This was not the high school sweetheart he had married. But the raw tears and overwhelmed feelings were real, and I could not hold it in. Have you felt like this?

"Is this postpartum depression?" he asked.

Up until the delivery of my children, I could count on one hand how many times I had tears I could not hold back. I am not one to be set off easily, and I have always prided myself on that. I learned later in life that being strong all the time is more of a defense mechanism that many of us learned from childhood pain. And we certainly do not earn merit points for defense mechanisms or for burying our pain.

I was not quite ready for the onslaught of tears and emotions that came as a new mother. I didn't feel overly sad. I felt tired. I didn't feel unable to cope. I felt overstimulated. The emotions would gush out of me even when

I did my best to contain them. This was all new to me, and I was not sure how to handle it or when it would pass. As a nurse, I've seen many women who have legitimate sadness about their new status as a mom; perhaps they were without much help or had other things weighing on them. I understand the tears and do not fault anyone for having them at any time.

Though I didn't have postpartum depression my first go-round, many women I know do and continue to have it after other pregnancies. I had what is known as the baby blues, a time of emotional upheaval characterized by crying for no specific reason and feeling overwhelmed. The baby blues is usually a temporary state lasting about three weeks where emotions are labile. This is due to all the hormones and life transitions we have been experiencing since childbirth. (Remember back when we talked about brain plasticity in chapter 3?) Let's look at this a little more closely so you can understand the differences between baby blues and depression, what is likely happening in your body, and what you can do about it, so you know, once again, that you are normal. Well, as normal as new moms can be, right?

Emotional Upheaval

Here's what I didn't know that I want to help you understand: When the baby blues last past the three-week postpartum mark or you begin to have more intense symptoms, such as extreme sadness or being unable to sleep, you may be experiencing postpartum mood disorders. Keep in mind that none of these feelings or symptoms are your fault. You did not do anything wrong, and neither did your baby. You are not a bad mother if new motherhood has kicked you in the rear. You are a normal mother.

Motherhood has a way of making us feel and experience things we simply never expected to. Even when we have heard stories from our friends about their experiences, we still somehow arrive with the expectation that we know ourselves, and we will not struggle in the same way. Sometimes we're right, and sometimes we're wrong.

So I looked back at my husband that evening and chuckled a little through my tears as I replied, "No, I don't even feel sad. I just can't seem to hold back my tears." I was so proud he asked me that question. Because here's the truth: Many of us women don't recognize our own signs of depression. We don't realize we haven't showered in a week or that we are overly withdrawn. It's common for our significant other to notice the signs first. Do not blow him off if he voices concern over the way you are behaving or feeling. He may be noticing something you can't see yet. There is no shame in having these feelings or calling your healthcare provider about them. In fact, I encourage you to call if you are struggling at all. They can assess your symptoms further and provide help so you are not in a downward spiral without a way out.

My good friend Ramona's experience was much different than mine. She, like me, was well trained and well prepared for what postpartum depression looked like, but she didn't expect to experience it the way she did.

Ramona felt numb and empty for weeks. She would hold her baby in her arms and wonder how she could feel so ungrateful to be a mom. *I prayed to get pregnant. I have wanted a baby for so long. What's wrong with me?* Ramona began to blame herself for anything that didn't go smoothly. When her baby would cry inconsolably, she assumed that it must be her fault. When she herself would sob, she decided she just wasn't made to be a mom. Feeling so sad at first slowly turned into not feeling anything. She simply moved through the motions day in and day out.

Ramona's husband, John, looked at her one day and said, "You don't seem like yourself. Do you want me to take the baby for a bit?" She replied, "I don't care." He asked, "Do you want something to eat?" She once again responded, "I don't care." John had her call her OB doctor who screened her for postpartum depression.

Depression, and other mental illnesses, are complex because we are multidimensional beings. We are spirit, soul, and body, and each one of these parts affects the other. It is not simply the signals in our brain that are at fault. Issues of the mind should not be treated as one-dimensional problems because the mind is not one-dimensional. Dr. Caroline Leaf, a renowned neuroscientist, states it beautifully: "Mind issues are being treated as if they were a disease like cancer or diabetes, but they're very different...These [issues] are intrinsically connected to our stories—our place in the world and how we perceive ourselves and others."[1] This is one reason depression is treated most effectively when we take a multidisciplinary treatment approach, such as therapy, alternative medicine, and medication. More on these in a bit.

I have a hunch that the neuroplasticity (the ability of our brain to reorganize and form synaptic connections) taking place during pregnancy and the fourth trimester is actually unveiling thoughts and beliefs we have carried with us for quite some time, maybe even all our lives. Throughout this motherhood metamorphosis, our minds are giving us the advantage of processing our world like never before. It is an opportune time to build our thoughts, mold our feelings, and become a healthier version of ourselves. You may not even know you need this type of rebuilding process, as I like to call it, but you are wise when you do work like this that will benefit you and your baby.

Ramona was diagnosed with late-onset postpartum depression. Postpartum depression is usually recognized at about three weeks postpartum, but for many, as for Ramona, it may be months before all the symptoms come to the surface. As she started medication and therapy, she began to notice a difference in herself. One day she realized, *I feel normal again. I feel better.* How long this change takes varies from person to person. Some women notice an improvement in symptoms within two days, and others notice after one month.

Depression medications are not magic seeds that grow instant, life-changing results overnight. They don't make you feel numb, and they don't suddenly make everything better. What they will do is begin to stabilize the chemicals in your brain so you can use the tools you know to use to help yourself. Depression medication is simply a tool you use when you need help to grab the other tools in your toolbox. It is a bridge that leads us toward healing. And at times it is necessary. Release any shame you may feel over needing these tools and remember that you are worthy of being cared for.

I often encourage mothers who are unsure if they have depression to speak with a safe, trusted person and ask them if they have noticed changes. This may be your spouse, a relative, or a friend. It's important to note that spouses may "blow off" your symptoms because of a false belief that your feelings reflect poorly on their performance in this new season. If your feedback is "This isn't a big deal. You'll be okay," but you know something's off, call your healthcare provider anyway. At times, we must be our own advocates.

Emotional Retrieval: How to Start Managing Our Emotions

Once you feel more aware of your emotions, you will feel more like a manager of them. I am a firm believer that small, simple steps can cause massive changes. Things don't always have to be complicated to be effective. As new mothers, we don't have time for the complicated. Some of the largest breakthroughs I received while processing emotions were with the three exercises I have listed below. First we'll ask ourselves, "What am I feeling right now?" Second we'll ask ourselves, "What do I need?" And third, we'll do a five-minute-per-day intentionality challenge.

"What Am I Feeling Right Now?"

This is an incredibly powerful question you can ask yourself each day. Motherhood can feel much like survival mode, but this question can pull you out of the chaos and put you back where you belong: in control of yourself. Do you have trouble pinpointing what you feel? A feelings wheel can help enormously with this.[2] I keep one on my fridge for this very reason.

With the neuroplasticity we are experiencing, we are quite vulnerable to new thoughts, emotions, and beliefs. Though this can feel overwhelming, with the right perspective we see that it is a time of great opportunity to look at what we are made of. This is a time when our brains are being shaped like never before. Old thought habits are surfacing, new thoughts are being birthed, and we are stepping into a new normal.

We can use this time of great transformation to stabilize our thought lives in a new way. What am I feeling right now? The answer to this question may be "overwhelmed, tired, stressed, bitter, hopeful," or other emotions. Whatever it is, simply identifying what you're feeling brings a moment of stability.

If you're not sure what you are feeling, that's okay. Look at the list of feelings I've provided and point out a few things that resound with you. Saying out loud, "I feel _____," tells your brain that your feelings are valid. Sometimes simply talking out our feelings makes us instantly feel better (that's one of the reasons talk therapy is so effective).

········ HOW DO I FEEL? ··················

· Joyful	· Sad	· Angry
· Content	· Lonely	· Bitter
· Peaceful	· Depressed	· Frustrated
· Hopeful	· Hurt	· Distant
· I feel _____.		

"What Do I Need?"

Once you identify what you feel, ask yourself, "What do I need?" It may be a nap. You may need to ask someone else to handle dinner. It may be that you need your husband to get up with the baby the next time they wake up. Sometimes you need something huge, but more often than not, it's a small thing that could make a world of difference. But if we are honest, we may wrestle with guilt and shame for even asking.

But I should be able to handle this. It's a common thought, and it is untrue. Every single one of us needs help at times. We were made for community. We were created to do life together and be dependent, to an extent, on one another. One of the first things God said to man after He created him was, "It is not good for the man to be alone" (Genesis 2:18 NIV). The word *man* here can be translated as "mankind or humanity."[3] Essentially, He was saying, "People need family." We can help usher out of our minds the belief that we should be able to handle this alone as we learn to bring in more healthy thoughts.

If you're having trouble identifying what you need, go back to the "What do I feel?" question. Often we can trace our feelings to what our need is when we don't rush past what our feelings are trying to tell us.

Five-Minute Intentionality Challenge

As you're learning what you feel and what you need, I want to encourage you to incorporate this simple exercise into your daily life. Take five minutes a day and do something you love. Ideally this would be when someone else assumes care of your baby, but I know this is not always feasible. Even if your baby is sleeping in a wrap on your chest, go ahead and give it a try.

Remember what you love. For me, it's putting my feet in the warm grass in the summer and looking at flowers or watching birds fly from tree to tree as I sip coffee. It could be going for a walk or drawing, painting a picture, or playing the guitar. It needs to be something that feels refreshing. Watching a favorite show or scrolling social media may work, but often these things don't actually make us feel alive. They're more likely to make us feel we have wasted our time, or we start comparing our lives to others'.

Five minutes doesn't seem like much (and if you can take more time, go for it), but the effort of being intentional in caring for yourself has enormous benefits. You matter. It's not just your baby that matters, or your spouse that matters. You matter. It's crucial that you not forget this just because there are so many needs pulling on you. You will bankrupt yourself if you continue to pour out but neglect your soul: mind, will, and emotions.

I encourage you to journal. Writing down what you feel, what you need, and what you did in your five minutes begins to develop core memories in your brain that pave the way for joy and positive thinking. Research has proven that exercises like this remove toxic ways of thinking and lead to positivity and overall wellbeing.[4] We are literally organizing thoughts, uprooting patterns of thinking that don't serve us well, and replacing them with healthy thoughts and patterns for our lives. If you need some help getting started, see chapter 15.

Postpartum Depression

Different than baby blues, there are times our emotions and thought lives are more than we can manage and feel bigger than our lives can handle. When this happens, we need to reach out for help. Postpartum depression is real. It is not emotional upheaval. It is an illness that usually requires therapy and medication to overcome. Sometimes the chemicals in our brains don't operate correctly. Sometimes they don't reset the way they should after birth.

If you are feeling hopeless or that you can't face tomorrow, you need help. Ask for help. Call your doctor. You may need depression or anxiety medication for a time. That's why it's there for you. Even if you are breastfeeding, there is medication that is safe for you and your baby. Many women feel they are not a good mother if they have to ask for help. It's actually the opposite. You show you are a good mom when you ask for help. It means you are responsible and getting what you need so you can care for yourself and your baby properly.

It's much like the instructions we get every time we board a plane. "If the oxygen levels drop in the cabin, and you have a child with you, place the oxygen mask on yourself first, and then place it on the child." Why is this the rule? Because we are not good to anyone if we are not getting our own oxygen supply. To truly care for others well, we must care for ourselves.

Postpartum depression can render us unable to use the tools we know to use. We don't feel we can pray; we can't worship, we can't even ask ourselves: "What do I feel?" It's all too overwhelming. I knew I needed help with depression when I couldn't put together a grocery list. It was something I had done repeatedly for years, but at that time in my life, I literally did not have the brain capacity to do what I knew to do. This is a red flag. Get help.

Dads can experience postpartum depression too. It's not usually because of a hormone imbalance, but tremendous life changes and lack of sleep can cause a father to experience these same symptoms. Think about it—his life has turned upside down too. He suddenly has more responsibility, and many new dads feel as if the weight of the world is on their shoulders. They become keenly aware that they have a little one who is dependent on them. On top of that, the woman they love is going through so much. She is uncomfortable, and she is struggling. Some men feel helpless when a baby is crying or the mother is crying. They want to help but don't know how. And if we are dealing with postpartum depression and can't form words to express how we feel or what we need, our husbands may feel powerless. Keep communication open with each other.

Natural Methods for Aiding Emotional Health

Because we are spirit, soul, and body, it's important to take a wholeness approach to our emotional health. Consider things like natural herbal supplements, nutrition, counseling, and medication. Nutrition is incredibly important for the restoration of not only your body but your mind. The gut-brain balance is more connected than we realize. Making healthy food choices can give you mental clarity and boost your mood. At times, our diet is simply low on something, like vitamin D, which can lead to depression. Here is where a supplement would be beneficial. A great counselor can help us process our feelings and pinpoint what's really troubling us. Each of these approaches is beneficial and can be even more effective in conjunction with the other. For this reason, I recommend you assemble a team around you or a holistically minded healthcare provider.[5]

NATURAL REMEDIES FOR IMPROVED MOOD

- St. John's Wort
- Omega-3 fatty acids
- Ashwaganda
- Vitamin D

- Cod liver Oil
- Maca root
- Light therapy
- Earthing

When starting supplements, always introduce one at a time.

SSRIs

Selective serotonin reuptake inhibitors (SSRIs) are the first line of pharmacotherapy defense against postpartum depression. The highest risk of postpartum depression (PPD) occurs in the first four weeks postpartum, though women remain at risk for PPD until five months after baby comes.[6] Women who have experienced depression before are more at risk for experiencing it postpartum. The most common antidepressant prescribed for breastfeeding mothers is sertraline (Zoloft). It has been thoroughly researched and proven to work well for postpartum depression and is safe for a nursing baby.

Real talk here for a minute. Never abruptly stop an SSRI medication, even if you feel great and like you don't need it anymore. Stopping these suddenly can cause a rebound effect leading to more depression or emotional lability. There was a season in my life when I needed depression medication. Once I knew I was doing better, I weaned myself off over the course of two months. But knowing now what I do, I would recommend weaning over at least six months. Be kind to your brain and give it time to adjust to lower levels of medication gradually. Your healthcare provider can guide you in this.

NURSE'S TIP

Always check with a lactation consultant, healthcare provider, or pediatrician on the safety of a medication or herbal supplement while breastfeeding.

What if I don't want to take medication? I posed this question to my postpartum therapist, and she recommended something that has been on my radar for several years: microcurrent neurofeedback therapy.[7] This is a therapy that exercises our brain waves. It's personal training for the brain, if you will. This technique has been around since the 1960s but has evolved and been studied thoroughly in the last several decades. Research tells us this therapy helps treat depression, ADHD, anxiety, OCD, bipolar disorder, sleep disorders, PTSD, and addiction.[8] Professionals like Dr. Andrew Hill, with the Peak Brain Institute, and Dr. Caroline Leaf, renowned neuroscientist, tell us this treatment is possibly more effective than medication and a great alternative.[9]

Remember, you are not alone. Any hardship you are experiencing is not your forever, and you don't have to suffer needlessly. You don't have to make enormous changes to see results. Small choices make big differences. Take the first step in front of you. Start there so you can see changes and growth in the ways you need to see them, and you will be so proud of the choices you are making. I promise you this does get easier over time, but you can't get to a healthy future if you are frozen in today. Let your needs be known so you can travel the path you dreamed of for you and your family.

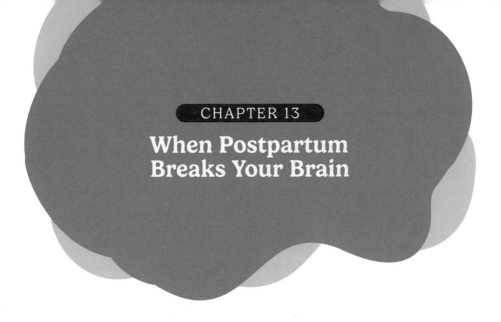

CHAPTER 13

When Postpartum Breaks Your Brain

S he had never felt like this before. As she held her baby tightly, she could feel her own shallow breaths, the tightness in her chest. Her hands shook as she changed her baby's diaper. She felt as if she may vomit.

She struggled to scroll through the contacts in her phone. If she could just call her best friend, maybe it would help. But wait—then she would know. Then everyone would know. *I should be a better mother. I should not be struggling*, she thought. She set her phone down and tried to focus on her breath.

Thoughts swirled through her head. *What will the night hold? Could we do this again? What if something happened to the baby? What if we don't make it?* The feelings of impending doom felt crushing.

Sometimes I don't even like my baby.

Wait, what had just gone through her mind? How could she feel this way? Tears began to roll down her cheeks. She cried out to God as she began to sob so hard she could not breathe.

Postpartum Anxiety and Postpartum Obsessive-Compulsive Disorder (OCD)

Postpartum anxiety and postpartum OCD often go hand in hand. Much of postpartum anxiety can present as intrusive, compulsive thoughts. This can feel very scary to a new mom and cause her to question if she's "losing her mind." Often, postpartum anxiety and postpartum OCD comes before the onset of postpartum depression.

A lot plays into this. From estrogen and serotonin changes to brain plasticity, much is happening in the brain. At times, dynamics in the marriage or family of origin issues also play a role in what comes up inside us during the fourth trimester.

Much like the new mom at the beginning of this chapter, my friend Nicole experienced postpartum completely different than she had planned. She was well trained and well prepared for what postpartum depression looked like, but she never expected to deal with postpartum anxiety.

Nicole had thoughts for weeks about getting rid of her baby. She knew something was wrong. She was not bonding with her baby the way she had seen other mothers do. She was told, "Embrace this time. It is such a connecting time for you and your new baby." But she didn't feel any of that, and it felt horrible. "What is wrong with me?" she asked herself over and over again.

One day her husband, Seth, looked at her and said, "I am not leaving you today. We are calling the doctor."

With an empty stare, she replied, "Why? You think I'm going to kill our baby?"

He replied, "I don't know."

She said, "I am not going to kill her, but I may give her away."

Seth insisted she call and refused to leave her side. He came to her rescue in more ways than she knew she needed. Nicole was diagnosed with postpartum anxiety with OCD. This was something she never anticipated, but she knew she could not handle her emotions on her own anymore. She needed medication and therapy.

Nicole is an intelligent, well-educated woman who works full time, educates others, and volunteers in her community. Postpartum disorders are no respecter of persons. It doesn't matter if you have a bachelor's degree or didn't graduate high school. And there is no one-size-fits-all treatment either, so it's important to be open to what your healthcare provider recommends for you.

After several weeks of medication and therapy, Nicole began to feel like herself again. The anxiety and intrusive thoughts didn't instantly disappear, but the days began to look more and more hopeful. She began to look forward to life again—to going out with friends and going to church. She could take her baby to the park, and she noticed the beauty of nature again. She noticed her baby's smile and how one corner of her mouth would rise more than the other. She noticed the deep red color of the roses wrapped around her fence. *How could I have not noticed all this until now?* she thought.

You are not any less of a good mother, or a Christian, if you deal with postpartum anxiety.

I hope you read that and let it sink in. I can't tell you how many new mothers deal with anxiety and feel something must be wrong with their faith or that they are somehow permanently flawed. Some have even wrongfully been told by well-meaning people that if they were praying harder, they wouldn't be dealing with such a thing.

This is completely untrue.

The fact that so many new mothers experience this convinced me I needed to bring a good set of tools with me to this chapter. My friend and postpartum therapist Tammy Bond also saw the need for this and helped put together the list below for you. I recommend you get therapy for yourself, but if that's unattainable in your life right now, start where you can. And remember, some therapy is better than no therapy. Even a session or two will help.

Tools for Overcoming Postpartum Anxiety and OCD

Anxiety and OCD can present similarly. Anxiety alone may come with intrusive thoughts but can also be more of a generalized, non-specific feeling. Rumination on anxious or intrusive thoughts or not being able to dismiss a single thought can become OCD, especially when you find yourself with a repetitive behavior you feel driven to perform in response to the thought. OCD symptoms are often quite time-consuming and cause impairment in day-to-day functioning.

- Differentiate yourself from the anxious or OCD thought. Do not create dialogue with the thought by saying, "Oh, you would never do that." Identify it for what it is. "This is an anxious (or OCD) thought."

- Find your essential truths. Identify what the truth is for you and use it to fight this battle. It may be, *I am a safe mom, and this is not permanent.*

- Journal. This helps you process your experiences and feelings. Have a tool to help you think outside of yourself, like a guided journal. When we see or write the intrusive thought or obsession, it can break its hold on us.

- Get talk therapy. A great therapist is such an asset! They can help you identify what's going on, as well as help you separate yourself from the intrusive thoughts. They will also help create a path that will lead to wellness.

- Consider SSRIs. This is one of the first lines of defense for postpartum mood disorders, and sometimes these medications are needed. Anxiety and depression usually go hand in hand, and these medications help both. It doesn't mean you will need it forever. It's simply a bridge to healing. (For a deeper dive into SSRIs, see chapter 12.)

- Look into microcurrent neurofeedback (MCN). This is a brain retraining system that exercises our brain waves. Research tells us this therapy helps treat anxiety and OCD, among many other things, by moving the client out of flight, fight, or freeze (the sympathetic nervous system) into our calm, clear, focused brain (the parasympathetic nervous system).[1]

Postpartum Agitation

Postpartum agitation comes from overstimulation or may be experienced as you are recovering from postpartum anxiety. Often mislabeled as rage, postpartum agitation is simply that, agitation. It often looks like becoming keenly aware of every single noise and touch happening around you. It can feel subtle, like your skin is crawling, or loud, like you are about to jump out of your own body.

Though you feel the agitation, pausing for a moment and leaning into body awareness can be a great tool. One of the first places I feel agitation in my body is in tight shoulders. For others it's their fists, or they may clench their booty. Turning your attention to your own body in the moment and purposely softening that area begins to put you back into body regulation.

When I began to hear the washing machine cycling through, the refrigerator buzzing, Peppa Pig's voice on the TV, the fan spinning on the ceiling, my son telling me he wanted a chocolate milk, and the crying baby in my arms all at an increasing volume in my ears, I knew I needed a minute. Noticing my tight shoulders and neck, I purposely softened them and counted to five. I fixed my son a chocolate milk and did it again. Soften the body and count to five. I could feel my nervous system beginning to calm down.

Postpartum Post-Traumatic Stress Disorder (PTSD)

At times we can experience a birth story that leaves us with symptoms of postpartum PTSD. I have worked with patients who have experienced this, and I felt it was important to highlight this disorder. Rather than going into details about their situations, though, I want to touch on how these moms experience this. Rage, nightmares, and feeling powerless or out of control are all symptoms of postpartum PTSD. Much of the time, these moms benefit from doing grief work with a trained therapist. Moving through the five phases of grief (denial, anger, bargaining, depression, and acceptance), as they are able, can help heal PTSD.

Retelling the story in a safe place is also powerfully healing. The story matters. It happened to you. And you matter. If you are unable to work with a therapist, journaling your story and then journaling it again can help you move toward healing. Perhaps this is the very reason complete strangers feel the need to unload their bad pregnancy, birth, or postpartum stories on mothers. Perhaps, for them, telling the story again helps them move through it.

ADHD (Attention-Deficit/Hyperactivity Disorder) and Postpartum

A dysregulated ADHD postpartum mom doesn't go about time management the way non-ADHD moms do. She doesn't wake up in the mornings with a list of tasks in her head to manage taking care of herself, her baby, and her home. Organization and scheduling are not usually on her mind.

Others around her may experience her ADHD as laziness or forgetfulness, but that's not true. The brain operates differently with ADHD. It's one of the best researched disorders in medicine, and here is what we know about new moms who also have ADHD: Close to 25 percent of moms diagnosed with ADHD will also deal with postpartum anxiety or depression.[2] This is important to know, so you can watch for these signs and get the treatment you need if necessary.

A few things that may help a new mom with ADHD:

- Lean on your support system. You may need a lot of help with the everyday tasks.

- Hire it out. If keeping the house clean is becoming an issue in your marriage, is it something you can hire out?

- Delegate the tasks that feel too challenging.

- If getting dinner on the table is a problem, can someone take on the task of cooking or ordering dinner?

At times, anxiety has been misdiagnosed as ADHD, especially for people who were diagnosed as children. It's important to get a professional assessment especially if symptoms are changing postpartum. Treatment may also need to be adjusted.

············

We all bring expectations with us into the fourth trimester, from the research we do to the stories we are told by friends and families. At times, our own expectations can derail us from what really works for us. I want to give you permission right now to be honest and say, "This does not work for me." I tell the story in chapter 6 of my own breastfeeding journey. I busted my butt to pump and feed my baby while running on a very low milk supply. I finally gave it up after months of exhausting myself. Looking back, I wish I had been able to give myself permission to do what was best for me.

When you are experiencing postpartum anxiety or other disorders and are trying to fit everything into the box of your built expectations, it can hurt you. Refusing help, therapy, meds, or simply choosing not to adapt to what realistically fits your needs can make your emotional state worse. Postpartum disorders can become postpartum psychosis (loss of contact with reality usually accompanied by paranoia, delusions, and hallucinations) when they are not recognized and treated. We want to avoid this at all costs, and we can do that by making changes when we need to. This could look like stopping breastfeeding or letting someone stay with you overnight to care for your baby so you can get a solid eight hours of rest. It is okay to say, "I know this worked for them, but this doesn't work for me."

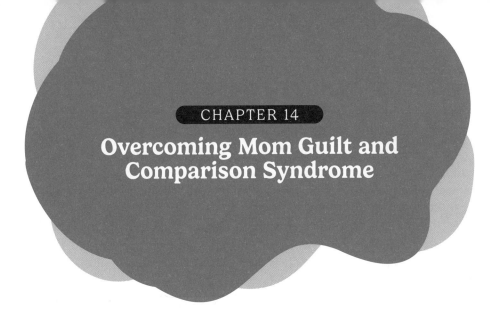

CHAPTER 14

Overcoming Mom Guilt and Comparison Syndrome

I tend to wear several different hats from week to week, and one of those is working as a childbirth educator. It's a role I enjoy because it gives me the rare opportunity to use my nursing experience and my parenting experience to help prepare new parents for their upcoming roles. I rarely teach a class without including this story.

When my son was eight weeks old, we started having a rough time. You may hear about eight weeks as "the eight-week sleep regression phase." Not all babies experience it, but it's a time when crying may increase and sleep may not be going as smoothly. It can last anywhere from one day to two months.

When it happened to me, I didn't know anything about it. In fact, only years later did I learn it was a thing. Even nurses struggle!

One day was especially tough. My baby seemed inconsolable. I changed his diaper. He cried. I fed him. He cried. I did skin-to-skin. He cried. I put him in his swing. Still cried. I took him outside. You guessed it, he cried.

I was out of options. I had no idea what he needed or what I was supposed to do. I had tried all the things. I finally sat him in his bouncy seat, sat on the floor beside him, and began to sob. He cried. I cried.

My husband walked in the room and asked, "What's going on?"

What came out of my mouth surprised me, "I am his mom. I should know what to do!"

There it was. The belief that I should be doing this mom thing perfectly, and that if I wasn't, it somehow meant I was failing as a mother.

It was a belief I didn't even realize I was carrying in my heart. I didn't say, "I am tired of his crying," or "I don't know what to do, and I feel overwhelmed." I automatically assumed I was failing as a mom because I couldn't stop my baby from crying.

I share this story with expecting parents because more than likely there will come a time when they are not going to know what to do. They may not be able to console their baby or figure out what they need. It happens to all of us.

Inability to console your baby does not mean you are not a good mom. I allowed moments like these to be judgments on my own worth as a mother, instead of aligning my thoughts with the truth. The truth is, I was a great mother, and I was doing the best I could—mothering is very hard work. It's also true that sometimes we don't know what to do, and that's okay.

When the thoughts pop up that you are not good enough or you should know what to do, it is important to remind yourselves of these truths to help overcome mom guilt.

- "I am a great mother."
- "I am the mother God chose for my child."
- "I am the right mother for my child."
- "God does not make mistakes."
- "God is more than enough for me in this moment."
- "It doesn't make me less of a mother if I'm struggling."

Pausing to anchor our thoughts in truth can be empowering in the moments we feel helpless. Taking the time to be intentional quiets the chaos of our minds and the situation and empowers us to become aware of our feelings and ask for what we need in a constructive way. Your communication with your husband may sound like this: "I feel overwhelmed that our baby is still crying. I need a ten-minute shower alone." And in the shower, you can remind yourself of this truth: *Even though I feel overwhelmed, I am still a great mother and am doing my best.*

Overcoming Comparison Syndrome

Never measure your own worth by another's opinions. Lord knows, I have done it, and it is a mistake every time.

When I was pregnant with my second baby, a friend decided to drop in for a visit. She expected things to be normal like usual, where we would sit down, chat, and drink coffee together.

It was anything but.

I had been sick for weeks while pregnant plus caring for my toddler, and I was doing all I could to simply get through everyday life. My house was a mess and my appearance...also a mess. My friend became frustrated with me and decided I needed a good lecture to get back into shape.

Of course, this did not go well. I already knew where I was lacking. Don't we all? I could see the dishes piled high in the sink and the laundry all over the floor. I knew the tub needed a good scrubbing and the rug a solid vacuuming. She thought she was helping me see the error of my ways so I could improve. But instead, it tore me to shreds.

Cue the spiral. I began to compare myself to all the other mothers. *They must be doing better than me. How are they keeping it together so well? I don't have a Pinterest-worthy home. It is not safe to show how I'm really struggling because others don't struggle this way.*

Here's the truth though: It's never wise to measure your own worth by another's opinion. And here's another truth: Someone else's reaction to your mess says more about what's happening in their heart than it does about yours.

My friend is not a bad person. She truly wanted to show me how off-kilter things were. And what spurred it all on was simply misguided expectations. I no longer had capacity for what once was normal in my home—sitting together and chatting over coffee. Not to mention coffee made me vomit in my pregnant state. In this season of young motherhood, things looked different.

She later apologized. And I accepted. We all have moments when we miss the mark.

It's so hurtful to compare ourselves with others, whether it's someone else doing it or us doing it to ourselves. Postpartum is an incredibly vulnerable time when we must protect our heads and our hearts. This may mean temporarily moving away from friendships that involve hurtful opinions and advice. It could mean changing your friend circle if you know they talk about you when you walk away. And it probably means putting some boundaries on what you scroll through on social media.

A couple of years ago, I was watching *Bluey* with my kids. Still to this day, *Bluey* is one of my favorite kid's shows. It portrays everyday family life in a beautiful way. In the episode titled "Baby Race," the mom, Chilli, is raising her baby, Bluey, and begins to compare Bluey's progress with all the other children's. An experienced mom notices that Chilli begins to withdraw and decides to share some truth with her: "There's something you need to know. You're doing great."[1]

I began to cry. This is what new moms need to hear. That they are doing great. That they are doing it right. I grabbed my journal and began to write. A poem poured out of me.

I want to end this chapter by sharing that poem with you. Anytime you struggle with your own worth as a mother, please return to it. Don't give room to mom guilt, a perfection mentality, or the comparison syndrome. You're doing it right.

You're Doing It Right

The dishes are stacked high,
The bottles left unsanitized,
You're doing it right.
The house a complete mess,
The laundry a wreck,
You're doing it right.
Holding your child tight,
While rocking through the night,
You're doing it right.
The days creeping…sigh,
But the years flying by,
You're doing it right.
Your hair messily piled high,
And feeling overwhelmed you start to cry,
You're doing it right.
Wrestling with feelings of inadequacy,
While overcoming others' shaming tendencies,
You're doing it right.
Giving it more than your all,
Not one sacrifice is small,
You're doing it right.
Because Mama, your love is much needed,
And in you, your child's heart completed.
You're doing it right.
So, when you question if it's enough,
Because this motherhood thing is so tough, remember
You're doing it right.

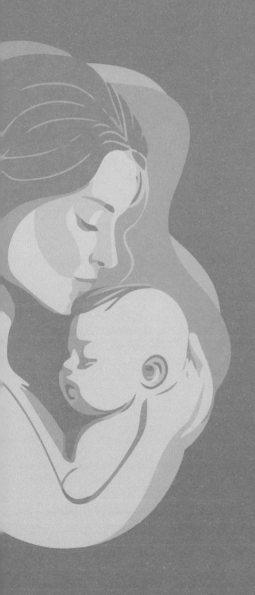

PART FOUR

Faith

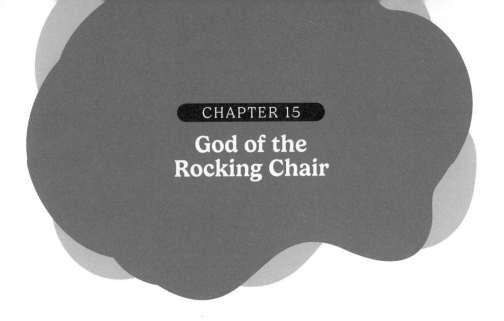

CHAPTER 15

God of the Rocking Chair

Time with Jesus looked different for a while after my baby was born. At first, I wondered if I was okay. Was it normal for my spiritual life to look so different with a baby in my arms? It was a Scripture verse here and there. It was a worship song I would sing while I rocked my baby to sleep. Connecting spiritually was taking on a different form. Did it mean I wasn't balancing life well?

It was unrealistic to attend a whole church service when the anxiety involved in getting me and my baby ready was crushing. I would get caught up in what others may be thinking of my tardiness and my up-and-down behavior during the sermon, and it paralyzed me. Then began the nagging mom guilt.

But here's the thing: When our faith takes a hit, so do our emotions and mental health. We are triune beings, made in the image of our Creator. And just like He is Father, Son, and Holy Spirit, we are spirit, soul, and body. And those three can't be mechanically separated from each other. If one is affected, the others are affected too.

Though our spiritual lives may look a bit different now, we still need times of connection with our faith. Our spirit needs our faith, our soul needs our friendships, and our body needs our care. We need care for all three to really thrive well throughout this time. To neglect one is to neglect the others.

So I managed to create little pockets of time to make sure I was not only attending to my physical needs, but also my spiritual needs. Asking my husband to take the baby outside gave me precious quiet time to read, reflect, and pray. And taking the time to journal grew a great spiritual connection to the Lord and served as an outlet for my emotions.

To answer the questions I had at the beginning of this chapter, yes, it's normal for your spiritual life to look different in the fourth trimester. You are now caring for another life on top of your own. But the Lord is beyond able to meet you where you are. He is not disappointed in you for being in a different season of your life.

One verse. One word. One line to a song. He has a way of piercing the depth of my heart and soul at the perfect time and in the perfect way. It doesn't take tons of time. In fact, God perfectly unravels my heart in a moment. He is the God of the rocking chair.

I have included some guided journal entries for you as a conclusion to this chapter. I've found that some moms have trouble knowing where to start with connecting spiritually again. In this new motherhood territory, things can look different. In time, you adjust; you find your routine and your stride again. But in the meantime, let the small steps guide you into connection times with the Lord.

JOURNAL

I feel

I am proud of myself today because

One thing I need today is

I want to remember

I have so much gratitude for

The Lord is my shepherd, I have all that I need
(Psalm 23:1 NLT).

JOURNAL

I feel..

....

....

I am proud of myself today because..

....

....

One thing I need today is...

....

I want to remember...

....

....

....

I have so much gratitude for...

....

Wait for and confidently expect the LORD;
Be strong and let your heart take courage;
Yes, wait for and confidently expect the LORD
(Psalm 27:14 AMP).

JOURNAL

I feel...

....

....

I am proud of myself today because...

....

....

One thing I need today is...

....

I want to remember...

....

....

I have so much gratitude for...

....

I am confident of this very thing,
that He who began a good work in you
will perfect it until the day of Christ Jesus
(Philippians 1:6).

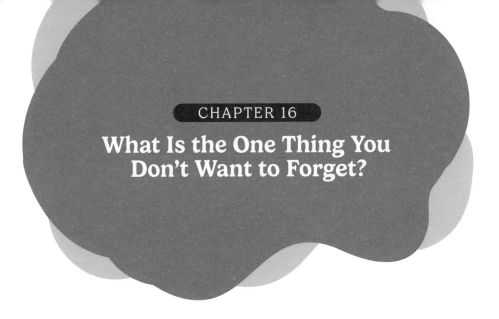

CHAPTER 16

What Is the One Thing You Don't Want to Forget?

Postpartum was tougher than I ever imagined it would be.

Between my body aching, exhaustion, a sore perineum, and sore breasts, my firstborn also hardly slept. It seemed he could not get content unless he could feel mine or my husband's skin. And a hand laid on him would not do the trick. He needed to feel our chests.

For months, at least five times a night, I was up. I was bouncing, rocking, singing, swinging, and swaying. Anything to get him to settle and sleep for just a little while. I joked often with people that this is how I lost my baby weight so fast. Though it was a joke, I would almost cry each time I said it. It definitely wasn't from trying to get back to exercising. It was from moving most of the night to console my little one.

I often wondered when he would finally sleep, and I heard different answers from everyone. Six weeks rolled around. Still the same. Eight weeks. Same. Twelve weeks. Same. Four months. Same. It was like an endless Groundhog Day, just like the 90s movie. I later came to understand that his love language is physical touch. Even as a small baby, he showed us signs of this.

One night, I woke up to his cry. It was time to nurse him again. I sat up on my bed, pushed the covers away, and took him into my arms. As I fed him, I whispered to the Lord, "God, I'm so tired." That was it. Everything I had summed up in one sentence.

Immediately, I felt His voice inside my heart: *What is the one thing you don't want to forget in this moment?*

I opened my eyes, lifted my head off my pillows, and looked down. There was my son in my arms. Fully content and at peace. His hand wrapped around my finger. How little it was compared to mine! My gaze turned to the rest of him. *Oh, look at how short his legs are. They barely hang off of my stomach!* I thought. *Look at his tiny feet. They are beautiful.* This was my baby boy.

He wasn't concerned if his mom would feed him or not. He didn't feel the effects of my exhaustion. He just felt peace knowing he was loved and given what he needed.

In that moment, I took him in with all my might. I did not want to forget this. I never wanted to forget how small he was, how his fingers would wrap around mine, or how he found complete peace in his mother's arms. I took a deep breath and sighed. Instant contentment.

I remember this moment so crystal clear. Though years have passed, and many memories have come and gone, this one stays with me. It's because in this moment, God reminded me to be intentional. He knew it was exactly what I needed to find strength in my exhaustion. To not rush through the moment, and simply be with my baby.

Many mamas experience exhaustion similarly. Some babies have their days and nights mixed up. Some moms work full time on top of being a full-time mother, so they rarely get a chance to catch up. Other babies have colic, the unexplained crying episodes that typically peak around eight weeks. Moms who have postpartum anxiety may find it hard to sleep even if their baby is asleep. They tend to startle awake at the faintest sounds or movements. Postpartum can be utterly and completely exhausting.

You are not alone. I see you.

Just like I didn't know what a charley horse was (a painful cramp in your calf muscle) until I was in my third trimester of pregnancy, I didn't know what exhaustion was until I was in my fourth trimester. It's a time when the days feel like weeks, but the weeks feel like days.

When things start to feel too tough to manage, pour your heart out to the Lord. Even if it's a whisper. Even if it's just tears. He can give us exactly what we need with one sentence. So Mama, I now turn this question to you. In this very moment, look around you. What is the one thing you don't want to forget?

....

....

....

....

....

....

....

....

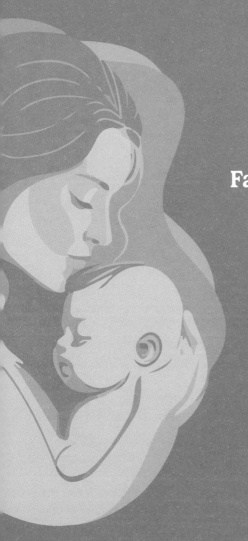

PART FIVE

Family and Friends

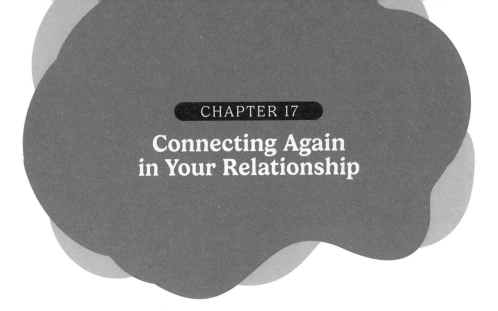

CHAPTER 17

Connecting Again in Your Relationship

A mama has been a mama long before she gives birth.

She has had many months to warm up to the experience of becoming a mother. She has seen her body change, felt her belly grow, and experienced her baby's movements. Whether she meant to or not, she has developed expectations of how this thing will go.

Dads have a much more cold-turkey kind of experience. It's normal for a man to walk into the new baby experience feeling a bit awkward and bewildered. He hasn't usually warmed up the way that she has. He's probably processing things quite differently than she is. It's common for a new dad to have more of a connecting experience with his baby in the delivery room than he has had in pregnancy.

We are different people. And perhaps nothing highlights that more than bringing a baby into the world together.

It comes as a shock to first-time mothers that many couples experience a negative downturn in their relationship after having a baby. Between the physical setbacks, exhaustion, and the strains of caring for a newborn, our marriage may suffer if we are not aware of how to manage it all. Few things will change our relationship like an addition to our family.

Though this is common, it doesn't have to be normal.

Communication

Communication breakdown is one of the number one issues in a marriage after baby comes. The stresses of recovery, the work of caring for a baby, and the transition into a growing family commonly bring with them the need to work on communication. I'm consistently taken aback by how few of us are taught healthy communication tools.

I certainly wasn't.

Night after night with a new baby had taken its toll on me. I found myself fed up and downright angry that nobody was helping me, especially my husband. *Can't he see I need help?* I would think, exasperated. Then I would assume he simply didn't want to help me. If he ever did ask, "Is there anything I can do?" my overwhelm would quickly make me answer "no," and he would believe me! Can you believe that? I assumed he should just know what I needed.

In reality, he was helping in many ways. Several times a week, I would go to bed early, and he would watch our baby until the first night feeding came, which gave me a solid couple of hours without interruption. But I still had so many overwhelming needs that what my husband would give felt like drops in the bucket of postpartum.

But I can see now that I never asked for his help. I didn't know how. In fact, I didn't even know it was okay to have needs. How could I expect anyone to do what I needed them to do if I didn't even know what I needed?

There's nothing like postpartum to shake up our soul and bring to the surface long-held belief systems. If our communication skills need to be tweaked, our postpartum relationships are sure to tell us. If we believe we should not have needs or are not worthy of being taken care of, those things come to the front during this vulnerable time.

Trust Cycles

We live with ourselves for so long that it's easy to assume that what's happening in our hearts is evident on the outside. Maybe you know what I mean. The truth is, it's our job to let others into our hearts. Yes, it's vulnerable and can even feel risky. But this is what creates true intimacy. A trust cycle happens when I express a need or desire, the other person responds to that need, meets the need, and in return trust and intimacy are built.

Even our babies are doing this with us! When our baby cries, they express a need, we meet that need (or at least do our best), and trust is built in the relationship. Not only that but meeting their need also teaches them they can express their need and expect that it will be met in a healthy way. We are teaching our babies from the very beginning what a healthy relationship looks like.

In marriage, it's important to give opportunities for trust cycles to be completed. If we hold in our thoughts, our feelings, or our needs, we rob our husbands of the chance to be there for us, and that in turn robs us of intimacy in our relationship. At times, we simply choose not to communicate because we want to avoid conflict. But failing to express what we feel is betraying our own hearts. The result will always be resentment and bitterness.

Past hurt often hinders us from expressing our needs and building healthy trust cycles. Can you remember a time you were vulnerable and it did not go well? What did that lesson teach you? Pain is a great teacher, but often it teaches us the wrong lessons. It teaches us to hide, to not express our needs, to keep our feelings to ourselves, that we are not as important as others, or that it's better if we just deal with it alone.

The first step to rewriting these lessons is to choose courage and express what we feel and what we need. Will our spouse always get it right? Unfortunately, no. But neither will we. Forgive, talk about it, and try again. Don't give up. Be like your new baby who has no reserve for being vulnerable, expressing their needs, and trusting that their parents will meet them.

Communication Tools

Hopefully, you walked into postpartum with a toolbelt full of healthy communication skills. But if you are like most of us, you didn't. Now is the time many of us first experience any kind of discontentment or conflict in our relationship. Or at least it might be the first time it bubbles up so much that it's impossible to ignore. We now have added pressures that we didn't have before, and this pressure reveals cracks in our foundation.

One of the greatest communication tools I have learned comes from Danny Silk, creator of Loving on Purpose.[1] It has everything to do with sharing what's going on inside me without shaming or blaming another person. We have all been a part of conversations when we immediately felt we had to defend our actions or even ourselves as a person. That's a terrible feeling, and we certainly don't want to bring it into the relationship that matters the most!

If we are on the defensive in a conversation, we are not bringing solutions. Our swords are drawn, and we're behaving as enemies on opposing teams. But this isn't our goal. We want to stay on the same team.

When something comes up, first seek to identify how you feel. Grab that feelings wheel (from chapter 12). Pick which feeling most reflects how you feel in the moment. To stay on the same team, incorporate this phrase into your vocabulary: "I feel _____ and I need to feel _____."[2] And then leave it alone. If you don't leave room for him to respond, you'll explain away or make excuses for everything you just said.

My husband is a dominant personality. If you are familiar with the DISC personality assessment, he is mostly a D.[3] These are great leaders, dreamers, and people who tend to change the world. They can also come off as abrasive or emotional bulldozers if they are unaware of themselves.

I, on the other hand am an S, a steadfast personality. I don't like conflict and feel that angry tones threaten connection. If my husband was short with me in his tone, I would shut down and emotionally disappear. But once we learned this was how I responded to his tone, we began to rewrite the scripts. In came the "I feel" messages.

One day I chose courage and connection and said, "Honey, when you use that tone, I feel afraid, and I need to feel safe."

The conversation immediately deescalated, and he said, "I would never want you to feel unsafe. That wasn't my intention. I'm sorry." Problem solved.

This conversation would have gone completely different had I said, "I feel like you are mean and such a jerk!" He would have immediately gone into defense mode and probably started shifting blame back to me (a natural reaction when someone feels defensive). We want to avoid at all costs the "I feel *like you* _____" messages. These are not the same as "I feel _____" messages. The first is a judgment on the other person's heart, and the second is a peek into the window of our own hearts.

Here are a few examples of healthy communication scripts:

- "I feel _____, and I need to feel _____."
- "Thank you for all your help. Will you _____ while I _____?"
- "I am so glad we are on the same team."

Feelings and needs are different, but you can almost always trace a feeling to a need. I shared with you at the beginning of this chapter that I didn't know how to have needs. I also didn't know it was okay to need. Because of this, I had to learn how to first identify how I felt so I could identify what I needed. Maybe you're the same way. I've found that many women, especially those raised in a strict environment, learned early on to hide feelings and needs in the name of being a good girl or behaving right. If this is you, here's a great place to start.

Begin to ask yourself these questions:

1. What is it you feel?
2. What is it you need?
3. What would be the most helpful to you right now?
4. Who may be able to meet this need?

5. Will you be courageous and ask them?

Anytime we begin to communicate differently, we face a learning curve. We won't get it right every time, and that's okay. It will feel awkward at first, and you may have thoughts like, *Is this even helping?* Every bit of work you put into figuring out what your heart is saying, and communicating that, will pay great dividends throughout your life. It is worth it, Mama! You are worth it.

When Gary Chapman penned *The Five Love Languages*, he created a revolutionary tool for couples. [4] Here is a quick breakdown of this tool. There are five love languages: gifts, physical touch, words of affirmation, quality time, and acts of service. Most of us have two main ways we receive love, and most of the time you can tell what these are because you tend to give love in these ways as well. If you are not sure what your love languages are, I encourage you to take a free quiz and find out.[5] It's much easier to send the "I love you" message when we know how our other half receives it best. It's also easier to tell them what we need if we are aware of our own love languages.

After you give birth, love languages can change. For years, when my kids were very young, one of my top love languages became acts of service. And it was no wonder! I was drowning in caring for children, along with a full-time job, household chores, and meals to boot. If someone wanted to show me love, all they needed to do was load the dishwasher or offer to care for the children to give me some alone time. Now that the kids are more independent, acts of service is no longer one of my top love languages. Love languages can shift in different seasons of life.

He Will Do It Differently

Mama, let me talk to you one-on-one for a minute here. Your husband is going to do things differently than you do. A postpartum mom will feel very vigilant over her newborn. She may feel that everyone is a threat if they don't do things exactly her way. Afterall, she is Mama. She knows best.

When my husband would hold our baby up in the air to get a smile, my heart would drop into my stomach. *Don't do that!* I'd think. My mom instinct wanted to keep my baby close to my chest and safe. But he was safe. Completely safe in his dad's arms. Dad played rougher than mom, but I wouldn't change that for anything now.

These postpartum feelings are instinctual within us in order to protect our babies at all costs. We were designed this way. This instinct helps shift us from only caring for ourselves to now caring for our babies. It helps our brains rearrange so we can prioritize the baby's needs, no matter how extensive they are—all day and night. If we are not aware this is happening in us, we can see the way our partner does things as downright wrong. This can lead us to completely take over caring for our babies, which can feel emasculating to him as the father. If we are not careful, we can altogether exclude him from this process. This only hinders his relationship with his child and can also cause hurt and bitterness in our own hearts.

Yes, the way he does it will be different. And that's okay. As long as he is safe and our baby is safe, we can allow this fatherhood process to play out. Doing so will only benefit the dad-baby relationship as well as give you help and increase the health of the family team.

Encourage him. Let him know he's doing a good job. I promise, he needs to hear it.

. . . .

The main advice I hear given to couples is, "Take more date nights." This is all well and good, but it can be impractical to implement with a baby. Personally, I don't think it's the lack of fancy restaurant dinners that causes our relationships to suffer. I think it's more in the everyday moments, conversations, and circumstances where we choose the other person, or we don't. Whether we choose to see them or not.

There are so many distractions. So much that draws our attention. The phones we hold, the social media we scroll, the games we play, the everyday life we do. One of the best gifts we can give our spouse is our intentionality. Our best efforts to see them, to hear them, to appreciate them, to show gratitude for what they do. I believe it's these moments that make or break our relationship.

So I will leave you with this challenge. What can you do this week to be intentional and promote connection in your relationship? Maybe it's a trip to a favorite coffee shop with baby included. Or it could be sitting together in the sunroom dreaming about a future remodel. Maybe it's being aware of the other's words of affirmation love language and saying, "Our baby is so blessed to have you as his dad. You are an amazing father." Whatever it is, I applaud you for taking an everyday moment and seizing the opportunity to be intentional.

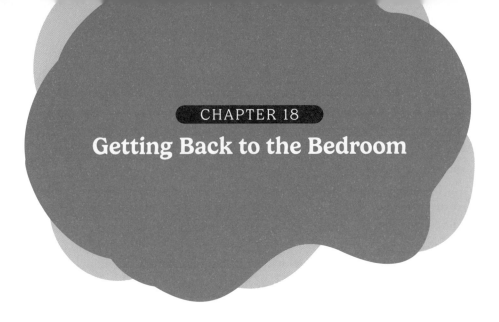

CHAPTER 18

Getting Back to the Bedroom

I knew the rule.

No sex for six weeks after having a baby.

Okay, no big deal, I thought. *Six weeks, and then it's, "As you were, soldiers."* I was in for a big surprise.

Most new mothers are told that they are back to normal at six weeks postpartum. At their appointments they are given the all-clear for sex, and may assume their bodies are just like they were prepregnancy.

Our culture puts a big emphasis on bouncing back after having a baby. I think at best this is an unrealistic expectation, and at worst, it's downright dangerous.

Thankfully, I had a great OB doctor. At my six-week appointment, she looked at my naive self and said, "Now, Rachel, six weeks is not a magic number. It doesn't mean you automatically feel ready to have sex again or that it feels normal. It simply means it's safe and you will not hurt anything."

I have so much gratitude that she gave me this information, or I would have thought something was wrong with me. If a first-time mother had a perineal repair from a natural tear or an episiotomy at birth (up to 89%

of first-time mothers do), her stitches are healed enough to have sex at six weeks, but her vagina and perineum (the area between the vagina and anus) may stay sore for several months.[1] Healing doesn't stop, nor is it complete at six weeks postpartum! Leading women to believe they should expect normal at this point sets them up for failure.

Even moms who don't have a repair or who have a C-section still need to wait to have sex. This is because when we birth our placenta, a large, dinner-plate size wound is left in the uterus. This shrinks and heals over several weeks. Our cervix also takes several weeks to fully close up again. Putting anything in the vagina while this healing process is taking place can introduce infection to our wombs. Ouch!

Some women don't expect to be any different after the birth. One nursing shift I was taking care of a sweet, young new mother named Lillie. I got her up to use the restroom for the first time and asked, "Did you bring any underwear?"

She said yes and had a family member bring them to me. As the extra-small sized red thongs fell into my hands, my eyes widened, but as reserved as I could I said, "Lillie, what do you plan to do with these?"

She didn't know what to think of my question and responded with, "Well…I'm going to wear them."

I held up the enormous postpartum pad that new moms wear and said, "No, you're not."

Now it was her turn for her eyes to widen, and she exclaimed, "Oh, I didn't know." I set out to explain what she could expect now. Turns out, she had taken most of her education from social media and thought she would simply bounce back after birth. She had no idea it would take her months to recover. The only pants she had packed were her pre-pregnancy size-two jeans.

Sex After Birth

The truth is that our bodies will continue to change past the six-week mark. Our hormones are also still shifting, and we may not feel in a sexy mood for some time. Breastfeeding also puts hormones into play that causes a decreased libido. So should we just forgo sexual intimacy until we feel 100 percent up to it? I personally don't think so. Sex is never just physical. It is emotional, spiritual, and should create connection and intimacy in our marriage. However, there is no reason to rush. Slow is your new sexy for the next few months.

There are ways to make things better for you, such as using vaginal suppository melts (looking at you, Femallay) or keeping a water-based lubricant on hand. Our lovely hormones may decrease our ability to naturally lubricate things for a while. Dehydration and the natural amount of fluid that goes into breastfeeding also plays into this. Talk to your man about all these things and let him know you are still healing. This is vital! We can't expect them to know if we don't tell them. They have also heard the incorrect message of, "Six weeks, and she is back to normal."

You may need to keep things more on the outside for several weeks as you continue to heal past the six-week mark. There are ways to have sexual intimacy without penetration. Incorporate this if you need to! Women with healing perineal lacerations that were minor may continue healing for months. Those who had major repairs (third- or fourth-degree tears) may continue to heal for a year. Orgasm is not going to hinder your body's ability to heal after six weeks, but rough penetration can if you are already feeling pain with sex.

Play around with positioning. When you feel ready for penetration, let him know to take it slow and go by your cues. He wants to be there for you, but he will not know what's comfortable if you don't communicate. This is a transition time, and it's not permanent. Intimacy may feel awkward, but it's worth it. Whether it's just cuddling time, outside intimacy, or full-on sex, every moment you spend together as one is needed for the relationship.

Body Perspective

Other things that may affect sex include our perspective of our own bodies. We are rarely prepregnancy size at six weeks postpartum. Pair that with leaking breasts, a shrinking stomach, possible stretch marks, and a stretched-out belly button, and our confidence may feel shaky. But this is not your forever! These awkward moments can create greater intimacy between the two of you. If your milk lets down during sex (and it will), laugh! Grab a tissue box and keep trying or wear a bra with nursing pads. One day you will be able to reflect on these stories and be thankful for the memories.

Some women feel concerned about how their spouse will experience their vagina after giving birth. As Rachael Elmore, my friend and couple's counselor of more than 20 years, states, "In all my years, I've never once heard a man complain about how his wife's vagina looks after giving birth. Hasn't happened. Not even once. I've heard them complain about every other thing. But they don't complain about cellulite, or stretch marks, or her being 15 pounds from her goal weight."[2] I've noticed this as well. Men don't look at our bodies the way we do. We tend to critique every little thing, but they don't (at least, healthy men don't).

As I wrote this book, I asked my own husband if he noticed any differences after the birth of our babies. He looked puzzled and said, "What do you mean?"

I got tickled and replied, "I don't know. Like did it feel different? Were you turned off by the fact a baby came out of it?"

He laughed and said, "Rachel, we are so deprived of sex after a baby that by the time we get to have it, we couldn't care less." It was a humorous but honest conversation.

Mom Brain

It's important to be aware that if you are trying to do the deed and your baby suddenly cries, your vigilant mom brain will kick in. It's incredibly hard not to go into mom mode instead of tigress mode when your baby needs you. Be sure to share this with your other half. They need to be reassured that you *want* to spend time with them, and this is a brain thing, not a them thing.

It was six months after my first baby before my perineum completely healed and sex felt normal again. Only after breastfeeding was done would I feel in the mood. This will vary from woman to woman. But this doesn't mean sex still cannot be fun and connecting.

If sex stays painful and doesn't seem to get better, or if things just feel really off after several weeks of trying, you may have some scar tissue or be dealing with birth trauma. Ask your healthcare provider for a referral if needed and schedule an appointment with a pelvic floor physical therapist as soon as you can.

Vaginismus

Vaginismus is when the vaginal muscles tighten up on their own, making vaginal penetration painful, difficult, or impossible. This can happen for all kinds of reasons: perineal tears or birth injury, anxiety, fear, or trauma. It can also be related to pelvic floor health. You are not alone in this! If you experienced vaginismus before birth, you may experience it afterward as well. It's best to make a pelvic floor physiotherapist consult. These are experts in pelvic floor health who can help improve vaginismus. Rarely does this get better without help, so make it a priority.

Dyspareunia (Painful Sex)

Dyspareunia is a blanket term that means pain during sex. There are all kinds of reasons sex could be painful, so it's not a diagnosis per se. Vaginismus can cause dyspareunia, but there is a reason it's happening (tightening of the vaginal muscles).

As you already read, painful sex (or discomfort during sex) can be common for a time after birth. Thanks to healing tears or episiotomies, along with possible scar tissue, sex may be uncomfortable for a short time. If sex felt good before pregnancy, chances are you are going to get back to that in due time.

If you struggled with painful sex before pregnancy and find yourself dealing with it again, make an appointment for a pelvic floor physiotherapy consult. Whether it's caused by vaginismus, a tight pelvic floor, or a weak core or pelvic floor, a pelvic floor physiotherapist can help you figure out the cause and get you a solution. You may find, with a little help, that your sex life after baby can be better than it was before.

Anal Sex

Though this used to be considered extreme behavior, anal sex has slowly crept into mainstream media, showing it to be a normal part of a sex life. This is not something I recommend to women on a normal day, much less when postpartum. We know from several studies that women, not men, are hurt the most by this form of sex. Because of our anatomy, anal sex leads to fecal incontinence, rectal bleeding, and anal sphincter injury.[3] Contrary to popular belief, we also know that anal intercourse has a higher risk of sexually transmitted infections than vaginal intercourse among heterosexuals.[4] Many doctors have been nervous to broach this topic with patients because of the fear of seeming judgmental, but women deserve to know the risks before making decisions about their sex life.

Intimacy Is a Journey

Getting back to sex was never meant to be a burden to us. The guidelines are not meant to rush us to perform. They are there to give you the permission you may feel you need to give your body time to heal after the birth of your baby. Knowing that sex is safe at the six-week mark, but also understanding that it may be uncomfortable or not feel normal for several months, is important so you can adjust as needed.

For us women, sex seems to be so much more than physical. It is connected to our emotions and feelings of connectedness and care in the relationship. If mama is overstimulated from being needed and touched all day, the thought of or request for intimacy can feel like another chore. Communicate with your spouse that you feel overwhelmed and let them know that being intentional with caring for you can add to the love tank. For example, "It would help me to be able to take a hot bath while you care for the baby."

Other ways to fill the love tank would be him giving you a massage, sending you off for a professional one, or rubbing your feet without any expectations of sex in return. When we feel cared for, it is easier to be intimate.

. . . .

I want to end this chapter with a return to one of the most famous scriptures in the Bible. In pop culture, it was also in Jim and Pam's wedding on the TV series, *The Office*. It's quoted so many times in wedding vows, even by people who do not consider themselves to be Christian. This universal truth about love rings true across many belief systems. First Corinthians 13:4 starts this way: "Love is patient. Love is kind." As you go about learning to create intimacy again with each other, I do not want you to forget the basis of what got you here in the first place: love.

Choosing kindness and patience with each other as you heal and recover is choosing love. Choosing it toward you is also loving yourself. What that looks like will be highly individual. It may be waiting another two weeks to have sex. It may be stopping mid-try and giving a back rub instead because of discomfort. It may be giving the other person the benefit of the doubt that they are indeed trying their best. There will be opportunities for bitterness to come in during this fourth trimester. I charge you, do not let it. Choose patience. Choose kindness. Choose love.

CHAPTER 19

Boundaries, Balancing, and Dealing with Unwanted Help

I f there's one thing motherhood teaches us, it's that balance is nonnegotiable. If we are to maintain healthy mindsets, we have to know our limitations. In the fourth trimester, much of our normal life takes a hit. New mothers tend to find their faith faltering, their friendships floundering, and their routines rooted out.

Let me raise my hand here and say, "It's me."

I was resentful at church. And I could not seem to keep my head above water at home. It's one thing to recommend to patients that they limit outside obligations, and it's another thing entirely to learn to do that for ourselves.

One day, I was hustling big-time to get ready for Sunday morning church with my toddler and second baby. My husband and I were on the leadership team, and expectations came with the role. Getting myself showered, dressed, my babies dressed and fed, and a diaper bag fully packed and prepared for whatever may happen is no small feat. And you can guarantee there will be a blowout before you walk out the door (the baby, not the husband), and you will need to repeat the process of dressing them all over again.

We were 45 minutes late for church that day. And the baby was miserable. I couldn't seem to get her settled. I wound up hiding in a small office space to nurse my baby the entire service. I left church that day feeling completely resentful that I had felt obligated to go. The bottom line was, I was not ready, and I should have said so.

It even felt difficult to schedule a bit of time with friends, but I was always so glad when I did. I needed that time to connect, process the struggles, and remind myself that there was indeed life outside of my home's four walls. Yes, I was a new mom, but I was still Rachel.

If you don't feel you have friends you can connect with during this time, I encourage you to find a mommy-and-me group in your community, a lactation group (many hospitals offer them), or a moms' small group at a local church. Even scheduling regular sessions with a therapist can help with this need. It is essential that you don't solely find your identity in motherhood. This will cause trouble down the road.

Necessary, Needed, and Not Now

It is for our benefit that we take time to decide what is necessary, what is needed, and what is not for now. Our first priorities are the necessary items. Our second are our needed items. And the not-for-now items are at the very bottom of the list. It's helpful if we can talk through these matters with our spouse too. This helps us come to decisions together about what daily life needs to look like. If we have a game plan for our routines, they will go smoother when the time comes. If you and your spouse are having trouble sorting through the details (which is common), I encourage you to take time and include outside help, like your therapist. It will help you simplify things for the long haul.

Necessary for me looked like sleep. With a firstborn that hardly slept, sleep became my number one necessary category. If someone wanted to help me, all they had to do was say, "I'll take care of the baby, go nap." Cue a deep sigh of relief! If an event or errand interfered with my ability to get rest, it had to be a no for a while.

Showering is an example of a task that could be in the necessary or needed category. Most of us new moms can manage going several days without a shower (though I hope we don't have to). For me showering was usually in my needed column, something I did once I managed to get a little nap and the baby was taken care of.

Not for now may mean not being able to hang out with your friends on the weekend until midnight because mama and baby will feel completely miserable. A great alternative would be to meet those friends for a lunch break between your baby's feedings. It may mean stepping down temporarily from a leadership role in the community or church until you heal more and find a routine. Here's the thing: We are still healing and adjusting way past the six-week all-clear mark we receive from our doctors.

Overcommitting and doing things only because someone else wants or expects us to will leave us feeling more drained and resentful. Not everyone will understand our decisions. And they may not agree. That's okay. It is not our job to convince someone else to believe we need what we need. Our goal is not to make them agree with us. Our goal is to communicate what we have decided, in the kindest way possible, so there is no room for miscommunication over the matter.

Netting, Electric Fences, and Elbows

Boundaries can look like many different things. If we want to keep birds out of our garden, we will drape a lovely green bird netting on the plants we want to protect. Sure, it's flimsy, but it serves the purpose and gets the results we want.

If my problem is black bears attempting to get into my bee boxes, bird netting will not do anything. When my husband and I visited Asheville, North Carolina, I noticed electric fences set up in yards around bee boxes. This puzzled me, since we don't have these in Alabama. My husband Dan said, "It's because of bears." Sure enough, we turned a street corner to see a mama black bear with two cubs walking through the neighborhood like they had just purchased a home on the corner lot.

At times our boundaries may look like bird netting and at other times like electric fences. And then there was the time that a boundary was a literal elbow. Dan and I were in Walmart with our new baby boy. He was in his father's arms and barely one month old. A woman in her fifties walked up to us and began to coo over our baby. As a new mom, my vigilant receptors were on high alert. But thankfully, my husband's were too. She reached out her hand to touch our baby. Dan side-stepped her. She tried again. He side-stepped the other way. She once more tried to put her hand on our baby's head. With one hand holding on to my baby's back, and one supporting his head, all Dan had left was an elbow. He threw his elbow up blocking her hand from our baby's face. The woman gave up and walked away.

Isn't this how boundaries can be? I like to think of my relationships as inhabiting concentric circles. God is in the center circle. The next circle out is my husband. The next out is my children. The next is close family and best friends. And so on and so on. The lines between the circles represent boundaries. Those closest to the center circle have fewer boundaries than those further out. By that I mean, the closer ones get more of my time and resources depending on the closeness and safety of the relationship.

After the birth of my firstborn son, my mom could give me a call and come over just about any time she wanted. I felt safe with her. I knew she was not judging my parenting abilities or the cleanliness of my home. She just wanted to be there for me, serve, and help with the baby. If there was a day that was not good for that, all I had to say was, "Mom, today isn't a good day. Would tomorrow work?" She always said yes without any guilt trips because her goal was to help. Boundaries with my mom are bird netting. They are flexible and moveable.

My dad was a different story. Our relationship was not the same. Because of some of his choices, he was moved back a few circles in my life. Further back equals more boundaries to protect my peace and wellbeing.

One day, I overheard him tell someone, "I go over to my daughter's anytime I want. I don't even have to call." I could feel the anxiety climbing in my chest. I nicely but firmly said, "No, Dad, you are welcome when invited, but I always need you to call before dropping in." I could tell it hurt his feelings, but this was required. He had not always made safe decisions. In my vulnerable state, I would not allow my emotional safety to be compromised. His boundary was an electric fence.

Check Your Intentions

It can be tempting when we first start setting boundaries to do it out of hurt, offense, or trying to teach someone a lesson. These are the wrong motives. Boundaries are to protect what's most important to us. They are there to manage the gates of our lives and keep the first things the first things. I didn't set boundaries with my dad because I wanted to hurt him for hurting me. A boundary is not to upset anyone or to please anyone. It simply is. It exists to protect what I have decided is most important.

It's always good before you set a boundary with someone (especially people you will be seeing on a regular basis), to ask yourself, "Why am I setting this boundary?" If your mother-in-law has been dropping in unannounced for weeks and is telling you how wrong you are for holding your sleeping baby, you may decide it's time for a boundary. Pause. Why do you want to set a boundary? Is it because unannounced drop-ins cause stress to your day? Or is it because you are fed up with all the advice and you want to "just show her!"?

A boundary put in place to hurt someone is not a boundary. It's a passive-aggressive tactic that stirs up offense and causes broken relationships. On the other hand, a boundary that helps you manage your schedule and peace of mind is healthy. It says, "This is what's most important to me right now, and I must protect it."

Tell Them About You

We get into trouble when we begin to tell others about themselves. We are all guilty of this. Phrases like, "You are so insensitive," or "I feel like you're selfish," don't show others our heart. They tell them what's in theirs.

I don't think we have the right to assume what's in someone's heart. Even if we choose to assume, who can truly know the depths of someone's heart but the Lord? Not only that, but communication often derails and crashes when we start telling others about themselves. Their automatic response is to defend themselves, not to engage or meet the need we have.

Make it a goal to tell them about what's going on inside you. We talked about "I feel" messages earlier in this book. These are great for helping you pinpoint those feelings and trace them to your need. They also allow the other to keep their defenses low because we didn't accuse them of anything. We simply showed them our hearts. They get to decide what they will do with that information.

If you have struggled with setting boundaries, here are a few things to remind yourself of. Return to these truths as often as you need them.

- They are valuable, but so am I.
- I will not betray myself by giving in to what is not healthy for me.
- Self-control over my boundaries creates self-confidence.
- I don't need others to approve of my boundaries.
- I will no longer do things simply because I feel obligated to by others.
- I don't control what others believe about me.
- I am only in control of myself and the choices I make.

Helpful Scripts

I was a classic people pleaser from childhood. Between my own personality that didn't like conflict plus an unstable living environment, I learned early on that it was better to appease and hide than show up with my own wants and needs.

For years in my adulthood, I worked to undo that harmful framework. But I literally had to learn phrases and scripts to help me communicate my needs and boundaries. It didn't come naturally because I certainly was not given those tools at an early age.

Sometimes, repeating scripts is what it takes. If you are not used to speaking what you need, or you have learned to go with the flow, or even if you have tried to communicate but your boundaries were plowed through, you may need to rely on scripts at first. It may feel awkward, but as you practice, it becomes more natural and even begins to sound like you! And remember, you didn't set a boundary to upset anyone, and you cannot control what they do. You can only control what you do, and you are choosing to build a healthy life you can be at peace in.

Here are some helpful scripts to guide you as you set boundaries:

- "I understand you want to connect. I do too, but right now isn't good."
- "I understand you want to connect. I do too. How about on (insert date)."
- "You would like me to ____, but I feel exhausted today. Let's plan for another time."
- "That question feels too personal right now. I feel uncomfortable sharing that information."
- "I've decided _____."
- "We talked about it and decided together that _____."
- "Thank you for the feedback. We will discuss it with the pediatrician."
- "I feel insecure in my motherhood when everything is done for me, and I need to practice my own instincts."

- "We need two weeks to recover at home before we will be ready
  for family or visitors. We look forward to seeing you then!"

Hopefully you never have a situation where your boundary is not
respected. But if you do, here are some possible scripts for that. Most of
these are versions of the tools from *Keep Your Love On* by Danny Silk.

- (When someone is angry with your boundary) "I understand
  you feel upset. I didn't decide on this to upset you, but I am 100
  percent clear this is what I have decided."
- (If they blame or try to guilt trip you) "That's a bummer."
- (If the conversation turns disrespectful) "This conversation
  has become disrespectful. I am happy to continue it when it is
  respectful again."[1]

Stick to your word—walk away until the conversation is respectful once
again. You control you, and if others want to be around you, they will learn
to control themselves.

Balancing and boundaries are a must in life, but especially in our fragile
fourth trimester. We can quickly become resentful when we don't manage
this well, and that resentment can stay with us for years, affecting our closest relationships. Being consistent and clear on what we need and what we
have decided will protect what is most important in our lives

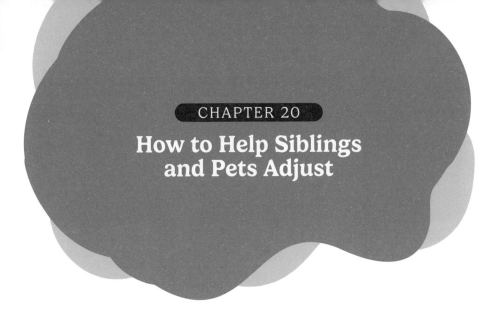

CHAPTER 20

How to Help Siblings and Pets Adjust

Most of the mamas I've cared for agreed that the biggest life adjustment they experienced was going from zero to one baby. Subsequent fourth trimesters were definitely trying, but most agreed that they were not nearly as trying as the first. This may be partly due to the fact that we already have a good idea of what to expect. Or it could be that we are more comfortable in our own ability to mother because we have been there, done that.

Whatever the reason, we are all thankful that it does seem to go a bit smoother after that first baby. But how can we help our other children handle a new up-and-coming addition to our family? This can vary depending on your child's age.

You know your children better than anyone else. What do they do around other children? Have they been around another baby? How did they behave? Use this information to form a plan for helping them adapt to a new little one.

NURSE'S TIP

Be sure to teach siblings about safe sleep practices for babies. Putting the baby to sleep on their back, using wearable blankets, keeping pillows and bumpers out, and allowing no toys in the crib is safest for baby.

Helping Siblings Adjust

Many older siblings will take ownership of "their new baby" when we give them roles to play in the care of the baby. We can teach them to brush the baby's hair, and when they do, exclaim, "Look how much she likes it! You are a great big brother." We can teach them the rules for holding the baby (with mom or dad's assistance). It's very important to make sure we are praising them for these things. Noticing the good and giving positive reinforcement will help cushion the times we need to correct.

To help prepare a young sibling before the arrival of the baby, get a baby doll or teddy bear and play "taking care of the new baby." Teach them to hold, comfort, and talk to the baby. You can even "show and tell" them where the baby will be sleeping and hanging out: bassinet, bouncy seat, stroller, car seat, or swing. Try not to panic if they hold the doll by the head or throw it into the wall. This is just an introduction to learning. They will understand a new baby is different than the doll once they meet them. Learning is a process. Having a new baby can be quite an abstract concept for a child until they experience it.

I felt sure that my two-year-old firstborn son understood the concept of a baby sister. He came to the hospital each day, held her, interacted well, and gave her a nickname, which forever stuck. It was after I loaded myself into the car at discharge and we were down the road, when he turned around, waved at the hospital, and said, "Bye Mon!" Uh-oh. Maybe he didn't get it like we thought. We laughed and pointed to the car seat beside him that contained his new sister, to which he had zero response. Thankfully, he adjusted beautifully even if there was some confusion to start.

Another important goal when parenting more than one is to make quality time for the older children. Are they used to going to the park with mom or going out for donuts on Saturdays? Make sure to plan some time for these things so they don't feel the baby is taking up all your time. This will prevent them from being resentful toward the new baby. It's tough to deal with seeing their mama now being shared with another!

When I had my third baby, I made sure we had a gift for my other two children in the hospital waiting for them when they came to meet their new brother. We told them this present was from their new brother. Technically, being in my belly made my decisions the baby's decisions. They loved this, and it helped them associate the new baby with a new fun adventure. Our oldest two still remember what their baby brother gave them the day he was born.

If once you get home you begin to hear, "I wish I was the baby," or "the baby gets all the attention," understand that they probably are feeling neglected. It helps to reassure them that you heard what they said, "I understand you feel the baby gets all the attention." If they are simply acting out by pitching fits, help them use their words by asking, "Are you feeling left out?" Young children don't have the ability to tell us everything they are experiencing. They can't say it; they simply feel it. We can help them by acknowledging their need, reassuring them of our love for them, and making one-on-one time to connect.

And to help them feel confident in where they are in life, when you take them out for special times, say, "I'm so glad you are two years old because you can eat donuts with me. The baby is too little for donuts." You may very well soon hear, "I'm glad I'm a big boy."

Helping Pets Adjust

Many mothers have fur babies long before they have human babies. These pets are a part of the family, and they are not expected to find a new home simply because there's a new addition to the family. Much like what I mentioned with other children, you know your pet better than anyone else. You know how they react around others. You know what they like and don't, so you are a wonderful resource for helping them adjust to a new baby.

A month before the baby arrives, begin introducing your pet to sights and sounds they will hear once the baby comes home. Turn on white noise machines, swings, and bouncy seats so your pet can acclimate to the noise. Begin using products you will use for your baby a little at a time. Occasionally wear a little baby lotion or wash your hands with a little baby wash so your pets can get used to the smell. If you will use special detergent on the baby's clothes, go ahead and wash a few items in it. You can also place these items in areas the baby will hang out most, and if your fur baby is a dog, go ahead and teach simple commands like, "leave it," and "stay" when they are around the baby's things.

NURSE'S TIP

Dogs and babies can have great relationships, but they should never be left alone together. Even when playing, dogs can get rough and nip. No matter how sweet your dog is, never leave them alone with your baby.

If you feel their routine will need to change once the baby arrives, begin to incorporate those changes one month prior to the baby being home. If your pet is used to being fed on the dot, begin varying those times so they can adjust to the change. You may also wish to invest in an automatic dog feeder if you feel this may become a problem. Cats will typically eat when they desire and are not on a strict schedule, so their routines are more unaffected.

Doggie daycare can also be a great option for the first couple of weeks after birthing a baby. It gives them time to play and socialize with other dogs and gives you time to adjust to life with a new baby. Other options are auditioning dog walkers before the baby comes, as well as planning a trip to Grandma's to be spoiled the first postpartum week. Go ahead and teach them on car rides not to get on the baby's car seat. This will help you anytime you need to travel with your baby and dog in the car at the same time.

For helping your dog meet baby for the first time, the American Society for the Prevention of Cruelty to Animals (ASPCA) states,

> It's crucial to stay calm and relaxed when you and the baby enter the house. If you seem nervous and jumpy, your dog will pick up on your feelings and may become nervous as well, thinking that the bundle in your arms is something to worry about. Instead, speak to your dog in a soft but cheerful voice as you walk into the house. Have your helper distract her with plenty of treats so that her attention is divided between them, your baby, and the other people present. The helper can ask your dog to respond to obedience cues, like sit and down, using the treats to reward her polite behavior. Praise your dog for any calm interest in the baby. Avoid scolding your dog. Remember, you want her to associate the baby with good things, not your displeasure.[1]

I also recommend that while you are still in the birthing center or hospital, after giving birth, send one of the blankets the baby has been wearing home with your significant other. This will allow your pet to begin to adjust to the smell of the new baby. You could even wrap it around a doll or stuffed animal and hold it the way you will your baby, so they get an idea of the new transition.

Never let a pet share a bed with your new baby. To reduce the risk of sudden infant death syndrome in babies, they need a separate sleep place away from pets, stuffed animals, thick blankets, pillows, or bumper pads.

Keeping your pet out of the room could also eliminate pet dander or flya-way fur that could find its way to your newborn's nose or mouth. For cats, placing aluminum foil on surfaces that are exclusively for your baby can deter them from trying them out. Supervised time together will give your fur baby a great opportunity to get to know and love their human sibling. In time, most pets adjust to the new family addition without any trouble.

············

It's always a bit of transition when growing your family. There are new routines to learn, and people or pets have to adjust to a new way of life. With some preparation, these transitions usually go smoothly. Patience and lots of grace will send the message to everyone that Mama is not worried about it, and they don't have to be either. Soon enough, all the members of the family won't remember a time when the new baby wasn't a part of it all.

Motherhood in Metamorphosis

*"Arise, shine, for your light has come,
and the glory of the LORD has risen upon you."*

ISAIAH 60:1

At the beginning of this book, I mentioned the metamorphosis of a butterfly, one of the great transitions we are aware of taking place in nature. That's us.

Our life prebaby is our caterpillar life. Valuable. Honored. We would not be who we are today without it.

And our life afterward is our butterfly life. Such a challenge to break forth from the cocoon of postpartum, but oh when we do, we are made to soar!

Postpartum is a shaking and awakening. It was meant to be. It shifts who we were into who we are. It plants our feet on a journey of motherhood. And even more than that, a journey toward more of who we are as women.

I remind you of this because it's easy to lose yourself in the cocoon of early motherhood. Unknowingly, many of us have been disconnected from ourselves for some time. We fall in love, and we dream about being engaged. We get engaged, and we dream about the wedding and honeymoon. We get married, and we dream about a family. We have a family, and we dream about...what? I think at some point, the whirlwind of our experiences caused us to miss out on some of the journey. I don't want that for me or for you. Doing the body, soul, and spirit work of knowing and caring for yourself in this time can allow you to be present and love wholeheartedly for every season of your life.

Let's not forget that postpartum lasts far beyond six weeks. Though some mothers feel more normal at three months, plenty of research (and mothers) shows us that the changes of postpartum can last for two years.[1] So please don't compare your journey to another mother's. There's a whole host of reasons you may feel normal sooner than her or she may feel normal sooner than you. None of it is right or wrong. It just is.

One morning as I walked around my backyard, my six-year-old son called my attention to something he could not quite identify. I couldn't believe my eyes. It was an imperial moth who had just broken free of its pupa (its version of a cocoon) and was emerging from the ground to fly. I softly cried because I knew the Lord was speaking some personal things to me and for this book you are holding. I watched the moth struggle to find its footing. But then it did what I knew it was designed to do. It made it. It did not give up. It broke free and went on its way. You will too.

I'm reminded of a thought I had one morning as I headed in to work for a 12-hour shift. I looked at the early sunrise in front of me and noticed blue and pink streaks begin to light up the dawn. I was in awe. I'm sure it's a coincidence that we have traditionally celebrated the birth of babies with blue or pink. But I see more to it. As I drove to work that early morning, about to welcome the birth of new little ones to the world, I felt God was doing the same. Painting the sky each day as a reminder of the glory of new life and new motherhood.

I hope I have provided a framework of grace, healing, encouragement, and understanding to the many things you experience in the fourth trimester. When you are tempted to quit, quit…but just for a moment. And then begin again. Be patient with yourself. You will learn to soar. You were made for this. Called to motherhood.

You are going to make it. And never forget, you are already a good mom.

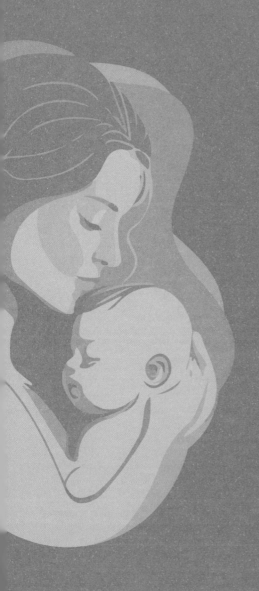

ADDITIONAL
RESOURCES

Help! My Baby Won't Stop Crying

Most pediatricians agree that crying for up to three hours at a time is considered normal. It's important to know that crying usually peaks between two and four months old and will taper off afterward. It doesn't mean you or your baby are doing anything wrong. It's a season that will pass. If you are struggling to console your baby, run through the checklist below. Take breaks as you can and enlist the help of your support people if possible.

Do call the doctor right away if your baby seems to be in severe pain, is not acting right to you, has floppy arms or legs, or is blue around the mouth or chest. Always go with your mom-gut. If you feel you should call, call.

Baby Care Checklist

- Did you miss hunger cues? (Hands to mouth, smacking, turning toward the breast)
- Does their diaper need to be changed?
- Are their clothes wet?
- Are they cold? Touch the nape of their neck. If it's cool, they may need an extra layer.
- Are they hot? Touch the nape of their neck or take their temperature. If it's hot, remove a layer and see if they calm down.
- Is it gas? Bicycle their legs, try baby gas drops or gripe water, or lay them on their right side (always supervise).

- Are they overly tired? Skipping naps does not make it easier for babies to sleep later. It can actually interrupt their sleep cycles and make it more difficult for them to go to sleep.

Other Techniques

Have you tried the 5 S's? The 5 S's were developed by Dr. Harvey Karp and work well for soothing babies.[1] First try swaddling snugly.[2] Once swaddled, turn your baby to their tummy or side (always supervise this time). This turns on the calm reflex. Now try making rhythmic shushing noises that matches the volume of your baby's cries while gently swinging and bouncing. White noise can also take the place of shushing noises. And finally, allow them to suck on the breast, pacifier, or a clean finger. Sucking keeps the calm reflex turned on in babies.

Most babies love to move. If you think about it, this makes sense. They went everywhere with mama for 40 weeks! As you walked around, it rocked them. And when mama finally settled in for the night, your baby started moving in the womb. It takes time to learn that stillness should equal sleepy time. Try baby wearing with a wrap or skin-to-skin contact. Babies are little sensory beings and love to feel the warmth and comfort of your skin.

Place them in warm water. Sometimes the sound of a running bath, plus the gentle, warm water can soothe a crying baby. Always supervise bathtime. Never leave babies alone in water, not even for a minute. You can get in the bath with them and hold them close. Allow the water to float around you.

At times, babies are simply inconsolable. This doesn't mean you are a bad mom. You won't always know what they need, and they don't know either! You are both learning. The good news is that they cannot hurt themselves by crying. If you have tried everything and are beginning to feel overly frustrated, lay them down in their crib or bassinet, let them cry for a few minutes, and take a breather. Take a shower or scream into a pillow. Get some of those feelings out, and then go back to your baby and try again. I promise you this will pass and there are better days ahead.

Help! I'm Having Trouble Bonding with My Baby

There are many reasons you may struggle to bond with your baby. If birth was nothing like you imagined or your baby needed interventions, it can shatter expectations you may have carried into postpartum. This can create disappointment and distance.

Maybe you didn't get to experience the golden hour with your baby. The golden hour is the first hour after birth where ideally a baby enjoys skin-to-skin on mom's chest. This helps a baby transition to the world gently and helps a mother get to know her baby.

When moms are unable to experience birth and the golden hour the way they anticipated, we know that feelings of shame, self-blame, and alienation can come into play. There are other reasons a bond does not naturally happen, like anxiety, trauma, fear of being a mom, or fear of repeating a parent's mistakes.

I need you to know something here. Maternal affection can grow. Just because you didn't feel it right away, doesn't mean it isn't coming. Here are some ways to strengthen the bond between you and your baby.

1. Hold your baby skin-to-skin often. This means placing them on your bare chest with them in a diaper. You can cover both of you with a light blanket. Babies are born knowing their mom's scent, taste, heartbeat, and voice. They are also highly sensory. Being close to Mama usually helps lower anxiety for them and helps them feel calm.

2. Breastfeed if you are able. Even if it's short term. Breastfeeding releases oxytocin that creates feelings of love between you and your baby. It also involves keeping your baby close. This produces the same effect for baby as skin-to-skin.

3. Interact with them. When they are alert and calm, talk to them. Look them in their eyes. Sing to them. Let them study your face. Let them hold your finger. It's important to know your baby is not rejecting you if they cry.

4. Be involved in their care. I know it can feel overwhelming to learn the *how* of all the baby things, but bathing them, diapering them, nursing them, and rocking them gives mothers a sense of bonding with their babies.[3]

As your baby grows, they will begin to interact with you in different ways. Small smiles, laughs, coos, and eventually reaching and crawling toward you all cement the bond between mom and baby.

If you have tried all these things and still are having trouble feeling connected with your baby, I recommend seeing a therapist. Fear or stress may be occupying the place of a bond. Now's a great time to find a safe person to talk with so you can overcome any shame or alienation you may be feeling in this.

You will learn this dance between mom and baby. Don't give up.

When to Call
My Healthcare Provider

The following are reasons you should call your healthcare provider right away. Always go with your gut, even if it's not on the list. If you feel like something is wrong, call. Your healthcare team would always rather you err on the side of caution than delay the help that you may need.

1. Bleeding that soaks a maxi pad in one hour
2. Passing large, baseball-size blood clots
3. Pain that is getting worse, not better
4. Headaches that will not go away
5. Blurred vision or double vision
6. Unusually high blood pressure
7. Burning the entire time you pee
8. Foul-smelling discharge from vagina or incision
9. Fever over 100.4° Fahrenheit
10. Excessive worrying or anxiety
11. Disinterest in caring for your baby
12. Hallucinations or losing touch with reality
13. Feelings that you want to hurt yourself or your baby

14. The feeling that you cannot cope with everything

15. Anxious feelings that leave you unable to function

16. Intrusive thoughts you are unable to manage

17. Any other reason that you feel you need to call

Other Issues

Though these are not issues every woman will experience, I wanted to highlight a few of these rarer complications because they always come with questions. I am sure you probably experienced someone sharing their horrible birth experience with you in pregnancy. This is never my intention, because the fruit of that is usually fear. Why induce fear of things that will probably never happen? That being said, I encourage you to dive into this section only if you are experiencing an issue that you have questions about. If you are pregnant, protect your peace, and read this only if needed.

Hernia

All the stretching and shifting during pregnancy can leave us more vulnerable to a hernia. This is when our tissues, fat, or intestines, push through a weak muscle and create a bulge. Hernias are usually painless (but can be tender) and you may notice them around your belly button, side, or groin area. Hernias can also happen around an incision for C-section patients. You may see the bump get worse when you cough, laugh hard, sneeze, climb stairs, or exercise. These are usually fixed by laparoscopic surgery. If you have surgery, give yourself time to heal well! Introducing exercise or lifting more than ten pounds after surgery too early can lead to recurrence.

Granulation Tissue

At times when an episiotomy or perineal tear repair is healing, it can over-heal causing too much new tissue to form. This can lead to an extra piece or dangly part in the area around where the stitches were. It may feel sore or cause pain with sex. This will usually settle on its own, but if it bothers you or is causing problems, make an appointment with your healthcare provider. This can usually be removed easily in the office.

Infection

It's important to keep the vagina, perineum, and anus clean as it heals after childbirth. Sitz baths and changing out maxi pads frequently helps with this. Rarely will infection happen if proper care is taken, but as with all things, occasionally it does. If you are having foul-smelling odor, thick, smelly discharge, pain that has gotten worse instead of better, or a fever, call your healthcare provider. Infections like this require antibiotics to heal.

Perineal Abscess

A perineal abscess is an infection that causes a painful lump in the area between the vagina and anus. It can happen after surgery in men or women, but with women it happens most often after childbirth (it's still a rare condition, happening less than 1 percent of the time).[4] Treatment for this may involve drainage of the area and antibiotics to kill infection. It also will probably involve follow-up visits to assess the healing of the area.

Skin Tags

These extended pieces of skin are benign growths that can occur in the vaginal area after childbirth, though they can form at any time, birth or not. They can look "stalk-like" and are usually less than half an inch long. They form in the folds of skin and are usually painless. Though these can be confused with an STI (sexually transmitted infection), skin tags often grow alone, whereas warts tend to grow in clusters. Skin tags are a normal part of change in your body, but if it bothers you, make an appointment with a dermatologist, who can help you figure out the best course of removal.

Bottom line, if you have issues with your healing tissues, do not try to solve it yourself. Check in with a professional.

A Note to the NICU Mama

Having a baby in the NICU (neonatal intensive care unit) creates a whole range of experiences for mothers. For a mom who had a high-risk pregnancy, she may feel relieved that her baby is now being cared for so intently by medical professionals. For a mother who did not anticipate her baby needing a NICU stay, she may feel taken aback by it all. Like somehow she did something wrong that caused her baby to need this kind of care.

Moms deal with it differently. Some of my patients grieve openly, ask me questions, and share their disappointments. And there are those who truly seem fine but are going through the motions of it all. Maybe everything happened so quickly that they were not able to process in the moment. Many times, grief will come later for these mothers.

I can tell you, though, the why of it all sometimes is left unanswered. Though we are forever thankful to have the kind of care the NICU provides, postpartum was not supposed to be this way. Never does a birth plan include a NICU plan.

It's okay to be a mess. It's okay to fall apart. There will be times you will, whether that's during the hospital stay or at home, weeks or even months later. Feeling incapable, anxious, worried, scared, sad, or angry can all be a part of this process. You will more than likely go through the phases of grief over several different aspects of your story. When grief is ready to come, let it come. Let those tears pour out of you as you process what was and what was not.

Can I encourage you to share your NICU story with someone? Telling your story, when you feel ready, is a great way to process the emotions of it all and move through grief. A social media NICU support group could be a good outlet for you. Though it can feel like such an isolating experience, babies are in the NICU every day. There are mothers all around you who have walked those halls.

If you find you are not managing your birth story well, talk therapy with a professional therapist who specializes in loss can help. Maybe you have not thought of your NICU experience as a loss, but a loss occurs when you do not expect this story. You are saying goodbye to what you thought birth, postpartum, and newborn life would be like. You may even be saying goodbye to what you thought motherhood would be like. That's a big deal. At times, because of the fragility of your emotions, hormones, and thoughts, you may need medication as you move through the fourth trimester.

Do not force yourself to feel okay. Give yourself the grace you need in the moment you are in. There is a light at the end of this tunnel. Though it's not supposed to feel this way, it will not always feel this way.

You are not alone. You are not less of a mother because your baby has a NICU story.

A Note to the Mom of Multiples

I often took care of mothers who had given birth to twins, whether vaginally or by cesarean. Some seemed calm and well prepared for the experience, while others looked nervous. As I helped one new mother latch one twin on one breast and one on the other, something dawned on me.

These moms are gifted a special grace to be a mom of multiples.

You have been through pregnancy, likely having to be monitored more than usual. You possibly carried extra risks and extra stretch marks, barely being able to shuffle forward as your babies' birthday arrived.

Those babies may have been skin-to-skin on your chest or had to be whisked away to the NICU for transition care. Maybe one stayed in your room, and one went to the nursery. Two babies. Two lives. Two hearts. One mama.

Remember to show yourself grace as you raise these babies. This first year may be one of the most demanding of your life. I know you are figuring out feedings as well as having to choose which crying baby to pick up first. It can feel completely unmanageable to have to get two babies ready and loaded in a car seat just to run to the store. Though at times it may feel you can't do this, you can, and you will. You are going to make it.

Don't forget in the midst of it all, you are exactly the person God purposed to be the mother of your children. Every one of your personality traits and even your faults are what God intended to use to shape your babies into the best version of themselves. No mistakes were made, Mama.

Take it one moment, one step at a time. Before you know it, you will be able to look back and say, "I made it! I did it!" and you will celebrate making it through your fourth trimester with multiples.

A Note to the New Dad

Having a new baby is harder than a fight in the Octagon. No, really. When you step into the Octagon, you know what's coming. You have trained for months. You have eaten the right meals, cut weight, and studied how your opponent fights. You are somewhat prepared for whatever the outcome, for there is a rhythm to this match.

When a new baby comes, it's different. What used to work with your person may not work for a bit. She may seem foreign in a way. Often emotional, anxious…different. I can assure you, she's still there. Her body and brain are going through enormous changes, but these will slowly begin to settle in. She may not be able to tell you what she needs. But she still needs you.

All these changes have a way of making a new dad feel powerless. When you feel you cannot fix her or even help her, or when your new baby is crying and seems to only want her, you may be tempted to think, *Why does it matter? I can't do it as good as she does anyway.*

Please don't step back. We need you. You bring a strength to this growing family.

Here's how you can help. Has your baby been fed? Take them out of her arms and tell her to go take a nap. Has your baby only wanted to nurse? Make or buy her a favorite coffee and clean a load of dishes. The smallest acts of intentional kindness will lift so many unseen burdens off her shoulders, even if she can't show you that.

Do not disappear. New dads can deal with depression just like new moms can. You matter too. Take a few minutes each day to reconnect with the person you love so much that you created a new life together. Ask how she feels. Tell her how you feel. Encourage her that she is the perfect mother for your baby.

A new dad can often feel unseen, but your role is more valuable than you know. Your baby needs you. Dads bring things to the table that moms cannot. We are different and are perfectly designed that way. Your deep voice brings security to your baby. The way you play and interact builds confidence. You bring stability and steadfastness to their life, even as a newborn.

So hold tightly through this transition. It won't last. She will find her way again. Find herself and yourself again. Her mojo will return as she heals and recovers. All in time and with intentionality, your relationship will grow close again and you will treasure these moments that are passing. Once again, you will find the rhythm of the match. Don't lose focus. Stay in the ring.

Index

ABDOMINAL BINDING, SEE BELLY WRAPPING

AFTERBIRTH PAINS 61

ALCOHOL 91

ANTIDEPRESSANTS 130

ATTENTION-DEFICIT/ HYPERACTIVITY DISORDER (ADHD) 138

BABY
5 S's/ calming your baby 196
bonding with 197
eight-week sleep regression 141
golden hour 197
hunger cues 70
safe sleep 186
when to call the doctor 195

BABY BLUES 122

BATH
for soothing baby 196
guidelines 63,91
sitz 33

BELLY WRAPPING 55, 66

BIRTH CONTROL 37

BIRTH
hormones at 29-30

BIRTH ACROSS CULTURES 13-17

BLEEDING
first period 36-37
postpartum hemorrhage 36
when to call your healthcare provider 36

BODY
odor 37
perspective 13-17
self-regulation 117

BOND, TAMMY 135

BOUNCING BACK 41-56

BOUNDARIES 177-184

BOWEL MOVEMENT 61

BRAIN PLASTICITY 28

BREASTFEEDING
bleeding or cracked nipples 74-76
breast massage 78, 83
clogged duct 78
colostrum 70
different size in breasts 83-84
engorgement 77-78
galactagogues 89
latch 67-68; 72-75
mastitis 81
milk supply 76-77, 80-83, 107-111
dropped 81-82
increasing 76
oversupply 82-83
night nursing 71-72

nipple shield 67

patterns 69

salt soak 75-76

tongue tie 68

weaning 83

BREAST SURGERY 76-77

BREATH

connecting with 48-49

diaphragmatic breathing 52

BURNING

incisional 60

while urinating 34-35

C-SECTION (CESAREAN SECTION)

helpful tips 63-64

therapies 65-66

CAFFEINE 92

CERVIX 32, 170

CLARKE, JORDAN 72

COLD THERAPY 31

COMMUNICATION

feelings 126, 164-165

in boundaries 183-184

preparing before baby 19-26

CONNECTION

with your baby 197-198

with yourself 117

with your spouse 167-168

CONTRACTIONS, SEE AFTERBIRTH PAINS

CORE 49-50

CRAMPING, SEE AFTERBIRTH PAINS

DADS

a note to 207-208

depression 129

will do it differently 166-167

DEPRESSION, SEE POSTPARTUM DEPRESSION

DIASTASIS RECTI 54-55

EMOTIONS

after birth 29

anxiety 134-139

grief 58

guilt 141-145

managing our rage 137

EPISIOTOMY, SEE PERINEUM

EXERCISE

5 Kind Movements 50-55

am I ready? 41-56

Kegels 46-48

walking 49-50

FIRST PERIOD, SEE BLEEDING

FIVE-MINUTE INTENTIONALITY CHALLENGE 127-128

FOURTH TRIMESTER 7-10

GALACTAGOGUES 89

GILMORE, EMILY 65

GOLDEN HOUR 197-198

HAIR LOSS 38-39

HARRIS, CHANDLER 31

HEMORRHOIDS 32

HERBS

for mood 129-130

in sitz baths 33

HORMONES

at birth 29-30

HYDRATION 92-93

ICE PACKS, SEE PERINEUM

INFECTION 202

INTIMACY, SEE SEX

ITCHING 32

KEGELS 46-48

LACTATION COOKIES, SEE RECIPES

LOCHIA, SEE BLEEDING

LOVE LANGUAGES 166

MARRIAGE, SEE RELATIONSHIP

MASTITIS, SEE BREASTFEEDING

MCNEIL, JEANNA 21, 93

MEDICINE
for anxiety 136
for depression 130-132
herbal for mood 130
with breastfeeding 131

MENSTRUAL CYCLE, SEE PERIOD

MICROCURRENT NEUROFEEDBACK THERAPY 131; 136-137

MILK PRODUCTION, SEE BREASTFEEDING

MILK SUPPLY, SEE BREASTFEEDING

MOMMY BRAIN 28

MORAN, RACHEL 34, 46

MOTHERHOOD
metamorphosis 191-192
overcoming mom guilt 141-145
truths of 142

MULTIPLES 205-206

NEUROPLASTICITY, SEE BRAIN PLASTICITY

NEWBORN, SEE BABY

NICU 203-204

NIGHT SWEATS 28-29

NIPPLES, SEE BREASTFEEDING

NUTRITION 87-94

OCD, SEE POSTPARTUM ANXIETY AND OCD

ODOR
body 37
vaginal 37

PADSICLES 34

PEEING, SEE URINATING

PELVIC FLOOR
exercises for 50-56
Kegels 46-48
physical therapy of 48, 65

PERINEUM
care of 31, 33-34
episiotomies 31-32
stitches 32
tears 31-32

PERIOD 36-37

PETS 185-190

PHYSICAL THERAPY, SEE PELVIC FLOOR

PLACENTA
brain, see mommy brain
cultural uses 15
encapsulation 36
wound 63, 170

POOP, SEE BOWEL MOVEMENT

POSTPARTUM AGITATION 137

POSTPARTUM ANXIETY AND OCD 134-137

POSTPARTUM DEPRESSION
Antidepressants/SSRIs 131-132
in dads 129
natural supplements 130
other treatment 130-131
when to call the doctor 199-200

POSTPARTUM HEMORRHAGE 36

POSTPARTUM PSYCHOSIS 139

POST-TRAUMATIC STRESS DISORDER (PTSD) 137-138

PREPARING FOR
POSTPARTUM
creating a team 23-26
rolling cart 23, 64

PROTEIN 88

PUMPING 78-80

RECIPES
drinks 98
meals 99-106
milk-boosting 107-111
snacks 96-97

RELATIONSHIPS
boundaries 181
communication
164-165
trust cycles63

REST
5-5-5 rule 44-45
sitting comfortably 32

ROLLING CART 23, 64

SELF-REGULATION
117-118

SEX 171-175

SALT SOAKS 75-76

SIBLINGS 185-190

SITZ BATH 33

SIX-WEEK RULE 42-43,
169

SKIN-TO-SKIN 197

SLEEP REGRESSION
141

STITCHES, SEE
PERINEUM

STRETCH MARKS 38

SWELLING 37

SWIMMING 63

TEAR, SEE PERINEUM

TWINS, SEE
MULTIPLES

URINATING 34-35

VAGINAL SHAPE 172

WALKING 49-50

WARM THERAPY 31,
77-78

YOU'RE DOING IT
RIGHT POEM 145

Notes

Introduction: The Forgotten Trimester

1. Eugene R. Declercq et al., "Listening to Mothers: Report of the First National U.S. Survey of Women's Childbearing Experiences," *Journal of Obstetric, Gynecologic and Neonatal Nursing* 31, no. 6 (November-December 2002): 633-4, https://doi.org/10.1111/j.1552-6909.2002.tb00087.x.

2. Carolyn R. Kline, Diane P. Martin, Richard A. Deyo, "Health Consequences of Pregnancy and Childbirth as Perceived by Women and Clinicians," *Obstetrics and Gynecology* 92, no. 5 (November 1998): 842-48, https://doi.org/10.1016/S0029-7844(98)00251-8.

3. Megan L. Aston, "Learning to be a Normal Mother: Empowerment and Pedagogy in Postpartum Classes," *Public Health Nursing* 19, no. 4 (July-August 2002): 284-93, https://doi.org/10.1046/j.1525-1446.2002.19408.x.

4. Harvey Karp, *The Happiest Baby on the Block* (New York: Bantam Publishers, 2015), 10.

5. Ferris Jabr, "How Does a Caterpillar Turn into a Butterfly?" *Scientific American*, August 10, 2012, https://www.scientificamerican.com/article/caterpillar-butterfly-metamorphosis-explainer /#:~:text=The%20caterpillar%2C%20or%20what%20is,which%20it%20sheds%20its%20skin .&text=Within%20its%20protective%20casing%2C%20the,as%20a%20butterfly%20or%20moth.

Chapter 1: Perspectives and Expectations

1. Joanna H. Raven, et al., "Traditional Beliefs and Practices in the Postpartum Period in Fujian Province, China: A Qualitative Study," *BMC Pregnancy and Childbirth* 7, no. 8 (2007): 1-11, https://doi.org/10.1186/1471-2393-7-8.

2. Catherine Pearson, "What the French Get So Right About Taking Care Of New Moms," Huff Post, January 17, 2017, https://www.huffpost.com/entry/what-the-french-get-so-right-about-taking-care -of-new-moms_n_587d27b4e4b086022ca939c4.

3. Sheetal Sharma, et al., "Dirty and 40 Days in the Wilderness: Eliciting Childbirth and Postnatal Cultural Practices and Beliefs in Nepal," *BMC Pregnancy Childbirth* 16, no. 147 (2016):1-12, https://doi.org/10.1186/s12884-016-0938-4.

4. If you are curious about postnatal retreats, you can see one option here at the Village Retreat Center: https://villageretreatcenter.com/.

5. William B. Ober, "Notes on Placentophagy," *NIH National Library of Medicine*, June 1979, https://www.ncbi.nlm.nih.gov/pmc/articles/PMC1807646/pdf/bullnyacadmed00120-0063.pdf.

6. Trisha Sertori, "The Unique Rituals of an Ancient Village," *Jakarta Post*, January 14, 2016, https://www.thejakartapost.com/news/2016/01/14/the-unique-rituals-ancient-village.html.

7. Olena Boriak, "The Midwife in Traditional Ukrainian Culture: Ritual, Folklore and Mythology," *Midwifery Today International Midwife* 7, no. 2 (2002): 52-4, https://doi.org/10.17161/folklorica.v7i2.3723.

Chapter 2: Prepping for Postpartum

1. Steven Covey, *The 7 Habits of Highly Effective People*, (New York: Simon and Schuster, 2020), 120-159.

2. See "Build Your Mission Statement," Franklin Covey (https://msb.franklincovey.com/) for an excellent, free mission builder tool.

3. Jeanna McNeil is a birth doula, birth and family photographer, and maternal mental health advocate. You can find more about her and By Design Birth Doula Services on her website: https://www.bydesignbirthdoulaservices.com/. This quote is from an email message to the author, March 27, 2024. Used with permission.

4. See https://takethemameal.com/ or https://www.mealtrain.com/.

Chapter 3: Your Physical Frame

1. Elseline Hoekzima et al., "Pregnancy Leads to Long-Lasting Changes in Human Brain Structure," *Nature Neuroscience* 20 (2017): 287-296, https://www.nature.com/articles/nn.4458.

2. Erika Barba-Müller et al., "Brain Plasticity in Pregnancy and the Postpartum Period: Links to Maternal Caregiving and Mental Health," *Archives of Women's Mental Health* 22, no. 2 (2018): 289-299, https://doi.org/10.1007/s00737-018-0889-z.

3. Barba-Müller, "Brain Plasticity in Pregnancy and the Postpartum Period: Links to Maternal Caregiving and Mental Health," 289-299.

4. S. Trifu, A. Vladuti, A. Popescu, "The Neuroendocrinological Aspects of Pregnancy and Postpartum Depression," *Acta Endocrinological (Bucharest)* 15, no. 3 (July-September 2019): 410-415, https://doi.org/10.4183/aeb.2019.410.

5. Copperstate OBGYN, "Adjusting Your Hormones Postpartum," Copperstate OBGYN, March 6, 2023, https://www.copperstateobgyn.com/adjusting-your-hormones-postpartum/.

6. Conversation with Chandler Harris, midwife (LM, CPM) on April 3, 2024.

7. Rutuja G. Choudhari, et al., "A Review of Episiotomy and Modalities for Relief of Episiotomy Pain," *Cureus Journal of Medical Science* 14, no. 11 (November 2022), https://doi.org/ 10.7759/cureus.31620.

8. Daniel Mota-Rojas, et al., "Consumption of Maternal Placenta in Humans and Nonhuman Mammals: Beneficial and Adverse Effects," *Animals (Basel)* 10, no. 12 (December 2020): 2398, https://doi.org/10.3390/ani10122398.

9. Miram Brennan, Mike Clarke, and Declan Devane, "The Use of Anti Stretch Marks' Products by Women in Pregnancy: A Descriptive, Cross-Sectional Survey," *BMC Pregnancy and Childbirth* 16, no. 276 (September 2016), https://doi.org/10.1186/s12884-016-1075-9.

10. Brennan, Clarke, and Devane, "The Use of Anti Stretch Marks' Products."

11. Claudine Piérard-Franchimont and Gérald E. Piérard, "Alterations in Hair Follicle Dynamics in Women," *BioMed Research International* 2013, no. 1 (2013), https://doi.org/10.1155/2013/957432.

12. Ablon Glynis, "A Double-Blind, Placebo-Controlled Study Evaluating the Efficacy of an Oral Supplement in Women with Self-Perceived Thinning Hair," *Journal of Clinical and Aesthetic Dermatology* 5, no. 11 (November 2012): 28-34, https://www.ncbi.nlm.nih.gov/pmc/articles/PMC3509882/.

Chapter 4: Strengthening Your Body Again

1. Rachel Selman, et al., "Maximizing Recovery in the Postpartum Period: A Timeline for Rehabilitation from Pregnancy through Return to Sport," *International Journal of Sports Physical Therapy* 17, no. 6 (2022): 1170-1183, https://doi.org/10.26603/001c.37863.

2. Jialu Qian, et al., "Effectiveness of Nonpharmacological Interventions for Reducing Postpartum Fatigue: A Meta-Analysis," *BMC Pregnancy and Childbirth* 21, no. 622 (2021), https://doi.org/10.1186/s12884-021-04096-7.

3. Beth A. Lewis, et al., "Randomized Trial Examining the Effect of Exercise and Wellness Interventions on Preventing Postpartum Depression and Perceived Stress," *BMC Pregnancy and Childbirth* 21, no. 785 (2021), https://doi.org/10.1186/s12884-021-04257-8.

4. The personal trainer I use is Jen Burns at https://www.strongerwithjen.com/, and my physical therapists are Emily Gilmore and Rachel Moran at https://www.thriveptal.com/.

5. Conversation with Rachel Moran, pelvic floor physical therapist, on March 21, 2024.

6. Bruce Crawford, "Pelvic Floor Muscle Motor Unit Recruitment: Kegels Vs. Specialized Movement," *American Journal of Obstetrics and Gynecology*, April 2016, https://www.ajog.org/article/S0002-9378(16)00035-1/pdf.

7. Rachel Selman, et al., "Maximizing Recovery in the Postpartum Period: A Timeline for Rehabilitation from Pregnancy through Return to Sport," *International Journal of Sports Physical Therapy* 17, no. 6 (2022): 1170-1183, https://doi.org/10.26603/001c.37863.

8. Yong-Sheng Lan and Yu-Juan Feng, "The Volume of Brisk Walking is the Key Determinant of BMD Improvement in Premenopausal Women," *PLOS ONE* 17, no. 3 (2022), https://doi.org/10.1371/journal.pone.0265250.

9. Marco A. Siccardi, Muhammad Ali Tariq, and Cristina Valle, "Anatomy, Bony Pelvis and Lower Limb: Psoas Major," StatPearls, August 8, 2023, see https://www.ncbi.nlm.nih.gov/books/NBK535418/.

10. A specific routine I highly recommend for preventing diastasis recti is Spinning Babies Daily Activities https://spinningbabies.ontraport.com/t?orid=142859&opid=26.

11. Menaka Radhakrishnan and Karthik Ramamurthy, "Efficacy and Challenges in the Treatment of Diastasis Recti Abdominis—A Scoping Review on the Current Trends and Future Perspectives," *Diagnostics* 12, no. 9 (2022): 2044, https://doi.org/10.3390/diagnostics12092044.

12. Anita Madison, Leah Bryan, and Laura Faye Gephart, "Prevalence of Planned Abdominal Binder Use After Vaginal Delivery," *Southern Medical Journal* 114, no. 12 (2021): 739-743, https://doi.org/10.14423/SMJ.0000000000001324.

Chapter 5: C-Section Recovery

1. Joyce A. Martin, Brady E. Hamilton, and Michelle J.K. Osterman, "Births in the United States, 2022," Centers for Disease Control, August 2023, https://www.cdc.gov/nchs/products/databriefs/db477.htm.

2. Benjamin Bleasdale, et al., "The Use of Silicone Adhesives for Scar Reduction," *Advances in Wound Care* 4, no. 7 (2015): 422-430, https://doi.org/10.1089/wound.2015.0625.

3. Conversation with Emily Gilmore, pelvic floor physical therapist, on March 21, 2024.

4. Ibrahim Karaca, et al., "Influence of Abdominal Binder Usage after Cesarean Delivery on Postoperative Mobilization, Pain and Distress: A Randomized Controlled Trial," *The Eurasian Journal of Medicine* 51, no. 3 (2019): 214-218, https://doi.org/10.5152/eurasianjmed.2019.18457.

Chapter 6: Breastfeeding

1. "Newborn and Infant Breastfeeding," American Acadamy of Pediatrics, https://www.aap.org/en/patient-care/newborn-and-infant-nutrition/newborn-and-infant-breastfeeding/.

2. This conversation with Jordan started in person, and she verified this information through an email on April 19, 2024. Used with permission.

3. I recommend the Talli Baby or Baby Tracker by Nara apps.

4. Frank J. Nice, RPh, DPA, CPHP, Mary Francell, MA, IBCLC. "Selection and Use of Galactagogues," *La Leche League International,* https://llli.org/news/selection-and-use-of-galactagogues-2/

5. Katarzyna Budzynska, MD, Zoë E. Gardner, PhD, Tieraona Low Dog, MD, and Paula Gardiner, MD, MPH. "Complementary, Holistic, and Integrative Medicine: Advice for Clinicians on Herbs and Breastfeeding." Pediatrics in Review. August 2013 343-353. https://www.ncbi.nlm.nih.gov/pmc/articles/PMC4530286/

6. Kelly Bonyata, IBCLC, "Lecithin Treatment for Recurrent Plugged Ducts," Kelly Mom Parenting Breastfeeding, August 16, 2023. https://kellymom.com/nutrition/vitamins/lecithin/.

Chapter 7: Postpartum Nutrition

1. Betina Rasmussen, et al., "Protein Requirements of Healthy Lactating Women Are Higher Than the Current Recommendations," *Current Developments in Nutrition* 4, suppl. 2 (2020): 653, https://doi.org/10.1093/cdn/nzaa049_046.

2. Sara Gottfried, MD, Instagram post, January 25, 2024, https://www.instagram.com/saragottfriedmd/p/C2iTBkhOjv7/.

3. Learn more about the dirty dozen list with "EWG's Shopper's Guide to Pesticides in Produce," https://www.ewg.org/foodnews/full-list.php.

4. Deborah R. Kim, et al., "Pharmacotherapy of Postpartum Depression: An Update," *Expert Opinion on Pharmacotherapy* 15, no. 9 (2014): 1223-1234, https://doi.org/ 10.1517/14656566.2014.911842.

5. Julie Mennella, "Alcohol's Effect on Lactation," *Alcohol Research and Health* 25, no. 3 (2001): 230-234, https://www.ncbi.nlm.nih.gov/pmc/articles/PMC6707164/.

6. Joan Younger Meek, MD, MS, RD, FAAP, FABM, IBCLC; Lawrence Noble, MD, FAAP, FABM, IBCLC, "Policy Statement: Breastfeeding and the Use of Human Milk," American Academy of Pediatrics, June 27, 2022, https://publications.aap.org/pediatrics/article/150/1/e2022057988/188347/Policy-Statement-Breastfeeding-and-the-Use-of

7. A. Nehlig and G. Debry, "Consequences on the Newborn of Chronic Maternal Consumption of

Coffee During Gestation and Lactation: A Review," *Journal of the American College of Nutrition* 13, no. 1 (1994): 6-21, https://doi.org/10.1080/07315724.1994.10718366.

8. I highly recommend Best Nest Wellness Mama Bird Postnatal Multi+.

9. I recommend Ferrofood, which you can find at Standard Process: https://www.standardprocess.com/products/ferrofood. It is also available through Amazon.

Chapter 11: Connecting with Yourself Again

1. J. Eric Gentry, PhD, "Tools for Hope, (Part II): Self-Regulation," YouTube, March 24, 2020, https://www.youtube.com/watch?v=a-75W_7sV7Y.

Chapter 12: Postpartum Blues Versus Postpartum Depression

1. Caroline Leaf, *Cleaning Up Your Mental Mess: 5 Simple, Scientifically Proven Steps to Reduce Anxiety, Stress, and Toxic Thinking* (Grand Rapids: Baker Books, 2021), 37.

2. This is the feelings wheel I recommend: https://feelingswheel.com/.

3. Strong's Concordance, "Lexicon: Strong's H120," https://www.blueletterbible.org/lexicon/h120/kjv/wlc/0-1/.

4. Karen A. Baikie and Kay Wilhelm, "Emotional and Physical Health Benefits of Expressive Writing," Cambridge University Press, January 2, 2018, https://www.cambridge.org/core/journals/advances-in-psychiatric-treatment/article/emotional-and-physical-health-benefits-of-expressive-writing/ED2976A61F5DE56B46F07A1CE9EA9F9F.

5. To begin the search for a holistically minded healthcare provider, ask family or friends for recommendations that lean into this lifestyle. Local midwives may also be able to point you in the right direction. Do a Google search for "precision medicine providers near me," "naturopathic practitioner near me," or "holistic medicine practitioner near me." Read reviews. A truly holistic-minded provider will listen well and take a multifaceted approach with treatments, such as considering gene expression, environment, blood testing, nutrition, supplements, and medication options.

6. Deborah R. Kim, et al., "Pharmacotherapy of Postpartum Depression: An Update," *Expert Opinion on Pharmacotherapy* 15, no. 9 (2014): 1223-1234, https://doi.org/10.1517/14656566.2014.911842.

7. My postpartum therapist was Tammy Bond with Wellspring Christian Clinic, Inc., http://www.wellspringchristian.com/Tammy_Bond.html.

8. Gloria Duke, et al., "The Effectiveness of Microcurrent Neurofeedback on Depression, Anxiety, Post-Traumatic Stress Disorder, and Quality of Life," *Journal of the American Association of Nurse Practitioners* 36, no. 2 (2024): 100-109, https://journals.lww.com/jaanp/fulltext/2024/02000/the_effectiveness_of_microcurrent_neurofeedback_on.6.aspx.

9. Dr. Caroline Leaf, "Podcast 201: How Neurofeedback & Brain Maps Can Help Treat Depression, Anxiety, Addiction & PTSD," Youtube, September 16, 2020, https://www.youtube.com/watch?v=1LVpOuzRInE.

Chapter 13: When Postpartum Breaks Your Brain

1. In person conversation with Tammy Bond on March 15, 2024. Used with permission.

2. Anneli Andersson et al., "Depression and Anxiety Disorders During the Postpartum Period in Women Diagnosed with Attention Deficit Hyperactivity Disorder," *Journal of Affective Disorders* 325 (2023): 817-823, https://doi.org/10.1016/j.jad.2023.01.069.

Chapter 14: Overcoming Mom Guilt and Comparison Syndrome

1. *Bluey*, season 2, episode 50, "Baby Race," written by Joe Brumm, directed by Richard Jeffery, aired November 17, 2020, on ABC Kids.

Chapter 17: Connecting Again in Your Relationship

1. See https://www.lovingonpurpose.com/.

2. Danny Silk, *Keep Your Love On: Connection, Communication, and Boundaries* (Redding, CA: Red Arrow Media, 2013), 101.

3. For more on the DISC personality assessment, see https://www.discprofile.com/what-is-disc.

4. Gary Chapman, *The Five Love Languages: The Secret to Love that Lasts* (Woodmere, NY: Northfield Publishing, 2015).

5. To take the quiz and determine your love languages, visit https://5lovelanguages.com/quizzes/love-language.

Chapter 18: Getting Back to the Bedroom

1 Ryan Goh, Daryl Goh, and Hasthika Ellepola, "Perineal Tears—A Review," *Australian Journal of General Practice* 47, nos. 1-2 (2018): 35-38, https://doi.org/10.31128/AFP-09-17-4333.

2. Rachael Elmore, *A Mom Is Born: Biblical Wisdom and Practical Advice for Taking Care of Yourself and Your New Baby* (Nashville: Thomas Nelson, 2023), 129-130.

3. Alayne D. Markland, et al., "Anal Intercourse and Fecal Incontinence: Evidence from the 2009–2010 National Health and Nutrition Examination Survey," 111, no. 2 (2016): 269-274, https://doi.org/10.1038/ajg.2015.419.

4. Emily Woodman-Maynard, et al., "Women Who have Anal Sex: Pleasure or Pressure? Implications for HIV Prevention," *Perspectives on Sexual and Reproductive Health* 41, no. 3 (2009): 142-149, https://doi.org/10.1363/4114209.

Chapter 19: Boundaries, Balancing, and Dealing with Unwanted Help

1. Danny Silk, *Keep Your Love On: Connection, Communication, and Boundaries* (Redding, CA: Red Arrow Media, 2013), 108, 117, 149.

Chapter 20: How to Help Siblings and Pets Adjust

1. "Dogs and Babies," ASPCA, https://www.aspca.org/pet-care/dog-care/dogs-and-babies.

Epilogue: Motherhood in Metamorphosis

1. Elseline Hoekzema, et al., "Pregnancy Leads to Long-Lasting Changes in Brain Structure," *Nature Neuroscience* 20 (2017): 287-296, https://doi.org/10.1038/nn.4458.

Additional Resources

1. Harvey Karp, *The Happiest Baby on the Block: The New Way to Calm Crying and Help Your Newborn Baby Sleep Longer*, Fully Revised and Updated 2nd ed. (New York: Bantam Publishers, 2015), 90-95.

2. If you need a swaddling tutorial, visit mamadidit.com/how-to-swaddle/.

3. Rose Coates, Susan Ayers, and Richard de Visser, "Women's Experiences of Postnatal Distress: A Qualitative Study," *BMC Pregnancy and Childbirth* 14 (2014): 359, https://doi.org/10.1186/1471-2393-14-359.

4. K. S. Venkatesh, et al., "Anorectal Complications of Vaginal Delivery," *Diseases of the Colon and Rectum* 32, no. 12 (1989): 1039-41, https://doi.org/10.1007/BF02553877.

Acknowledgments

S o many of you have championed this book. I am grateful for each of your contributions, whether it was an interview where you shared your expertise or encouragement and prayer you gifted to me as I wrote. With all my heart, thank you so much.

To Blythe Daniel, the best agent, who has been a beautiful gift to me. To Chandler Harris at Birth Right Birmingham Midwifery, Emily Gilmore and Rachel Moran at Thrive Physical Therapy and Wellness, Heather Jones Skaggs, Content Director at the Bluff Park Reader, Jeanna McNeil at ByDesign Birth Doula Services, Jen Burns at Stronger with Jen Personal Training, Jordan Clarke at Birmingham Breastfeeding, Madonna Nichols at St. Vincent's Birmingham, and Tammy Bond at Wellspring Christian Clinic, thank you for all your contributions and the way you uphold new mothers.

To my husband Dan, who gave me the encouragement and space I needed to pour out my years of experience into a book. I am so grateful for who you are. To my lovely children who have also believed in this book and found such joy in the thought of me helping new mothers and babies. You are some of the greatest gifts I have ever been given. To Audrey, Emma, and everyone at Harvest House Publishers for believing in me and the vision of this beautiful book. And to every mom friend who let me share her story or had long conversations with me about all they were experiencing, thank you!

About the Author

RACHEL TAYLOR is a registered nurse and childbirth educator who specializes in the care of mothers and babies. With more than 15 years of experience as a postpartum nurse, her passion is to bridge the gap between the current healthcare model and a mom's needs in the fourth trimester. Rachel is also the founder of Mama Did It, a nurse-written blog for a woman's journey throughout pregnancy, postpartum, and motherhood. She lives with her husband and three children in Birmingham, Alabama.